SOCCER INJURIES:

A Physical Therapy View in Care and Prevention

Soccer Injuries:
A Physical Therapy View in Care and Prevention

by
Harry Nafpliotis

VANTAGE PRESS
New York / Washington / Atlanta
Los Angeles / Chicago

FIRST EDITION

Published by Vantage Press, Inc.
516 West 34th Street, New York, New York 10001

Manufactured in the United States of America
ISBN: 533-04635-1

Library of Congress Catalog Card No.: 80-50386

131908

Contents

Acknowledgements

Material from *Handbook of Physical Medicine and Rehabilitation,* by Krusen, Kottke and Elmwood, 1968, pp. 23–8, is used by permission.

Material from *Athletic Training and Conditioning,* by O. William Dayton, 1965, pp. 199, 215, 309, 344, is used by permission.

Material from *Functional Anatomy of the Limbs and Back* by W.H. Hollinshead, 1960, pp. 299, 301, is used by permission.

Material from *Training and Conditioning of Athletes,* by Max M. Novich and Buddy Taylor, Lea and Febiger, Publisher, 1970, pp. 194, 200–1, is used by permission.

Material from *A Manual of Bandaging, Splinting and Strapping,* by Augustus Thorndike, Jr., M.D., Lea and Febiger, Publisher, 1941, is used by permission.

Material from *A Manual of Electrotherapy,* (2nd ed.) by Arthur L. Watkins, M.D., Lea and Febiger, Publisher, 1962, pp. 241–2, 251, is used by permission.

Material from *Anatomical Correlates of Clinical Electromyography,* by Joseph Goodgold, M.D., 1974, pp. 15, 19, is used by permission.

Soccer Week, Soccer Action photos, by Dennis T. O'Donnell.

Ridgewood News, Soccer photo action "A Kick in the Head" by Rich McBride.

Grateful acknowledgement is made to V. Estacio, C. Gaeta, J.D. Price, J. Meehan, G. Nafpliotis (son), and E. Walton, who served as models in some of the photographs for *Soccer Injuries.* A special thanks to Adria Rosenstein who contributed to much in modeling the enclosed photographs.

Special thanks are due to Dr. J.V. Cerney for the use of a number of illustrations and material from his excellent book *Athletic Injuries.*

Introduction: Brief History of Soccer

It is not certain exactly where, when, or how the game of soccer originated. There are several very different versions. According to one soccer historian, the game began about the time the Vikings attempted to invade Saxony. In order to celebrate the capture of a Viking, the Saxons would play a game of football, or soccer, as it is now called in the United States, using the prisoner as the "football!" As the game developed with time, the Saxons used only the head of the victim as the object of their booting, thus accelerating the pace of the game. This theoretically progressed to the modern-day game of soccer, using an inflated leather ball. Another historian reports that the game originated in ancient Greece and was at that time called "*Harpaston.*" According to this version, the ball was moved by any means across goal lines, which were usually at opposite ends of the town. A form of this ancient Greek game was adopted by the Romans, who used the sport not only for recreation but also as one aspect of military training. As the Romans began to conquer the lands that now comprise Europe, the game was introduced to these regions.

Regardless of its origin, soccer is at the present time the only true international sport. In many countries, it is a national sport. Its popularity throughout the world may in part be attributed to the Romans, who introduced the game of soccer (or as it is called in most countries, football) to the modern civilizations. However, the major credit should go to the sport itself for several reasons. Its simplicity of rules and strategy makes it easy for both the participant and spectator to understand. With proper training, even a novice can master the sport without too much difficulty. Age is not a limiting factor in soccer—the only prerequisite is conditional stamina. Playing soccer helps to develop characteristics such as coordination and self-control. Due to restricted use of the hands and limited body contact, soccer is among the safest sports played today. Little equipment is required, which makes the sport very popular at all school levels because it offers low budgetary financing. If necessary, the soccer player may wear ordinary gym clothes. The only other equipment needed is a pair of soccer shoes, shin guards, and, of course, a soccer ball.

Soccer became an organized sport in 1904 with the formation of the Federation Internationale de Football Association (F.I.F.A.). Originally, it had seven member countries. It has now expanded to include 140 countries in six continental confederations. The United States developed its own soccer organization, the United States Soccer Federation (U.S.S.F.), in 1913, but only two states participated. The popularity of soccer increased with the formation of the German American Soccer League (presently known as the Cosmopolitan Soccer League), with the involvement in soccer of such ethnic groups as Greeks, Italians, Germans, English, and Slavs. The major impetus for the growing popularity of soccer in this country has come in the past ten years with the formation of professional leagues, the establishment of fine coaching schools, the public relations of the American league and mostly of the big promoters of the North American Soccer League (N.A.S.L.). "Thanks largely to an influx of big-name foreign players and low ticket prices, the crowds at a number of N.A.S.L. franchises have sprouted to pro-football proportions," admits J. D. Reed (*Sports Illustrated*, August 1977). Who exactly is filling the stands around the country? Reed, continues:

> If you think that a typical N.A.S.L. fan is of European or South American descent and goes to a soccer match fondly recalling the same in the old country, you are wrong. The new American soccer crowd is not ethnic; it is middle and upper class, younger than an N.F.L. crowd (averaging 18–25), more than half college educated, almost half women and a third children under fourteen. Tampa and Dallas closely conform to this profile and in Dallas more than a third of the average crowd of 16,500 earns in excess of $25,000 a year.

We can not take anything away from Pele's contribution to the N.A.S.L. At the same time, we can not underestimate the youth soccer movement in the United States which has contributed to the game's new popularity. Finally, soccer is growing very rapidly in this country, and reports of its popularity indicate that it is here to stay. As Reed pointed out:

> You can market all you want but sports must follow people's moods, not create them. Soccer is the now sport . . . Like tennis, soccer has a great deal of individual creativity . . . it has a fluid

movement that fits the times . . . to make it in a major-sports market, not pushing anybody out of the way but filling a gap. . . . That's what soccer is all about. That's success.

This book is meant to be of benefit to the soccer trainer, coach, and player by presenting the fundamental principles of preventive and corrective measures to soccer injuries through the application of physical-therapy techniques. It is written with the intent of being as concise as possible, yet at the same time being in sufficient depth to cover the many aspects of the subject. The book represents a consensus of the theories and opinions of many authors and athletic trainers as they have recorded their ideas in the literature. The methods presented in this book are supported by the experience of several instructors of athletic training, physical education, and other related fields.

This book will hopefully clarify the point of who should be responsible for the treatment of soccer injuries. It must be emphasized to the soccer coach that his responsibility lies mainly in the prevention of soccer injuries rather than in the care and treatment of such injuries. Treatment should be left to the supervision of a medical doctor. It is unrealistic, however, to assume that the services of a physician or hospital facility will always be available to the athlete at the time of an injury, when immediate treatment may be crucial. An alternative measure to ensure such immediate care would be to have a physical therapist present at all practice sessions or at least at all games. In cooperation with the trainer, a physical therapist would be able to provide first-aid care and consult the physician should that be necessary.

During the past decade, soccer has become a fundamental component of the physical-education programs at all school levels as well as at the professional level. This rapid development of soccer's popularity should, in itself, validate the need of a book concerned with the care and prevention of soccer injuries. A book such as this will help to ensure the safety of the players themselves.

In describing the prevention and treatment of athletic injuries, the scope of this book is confined to only those pertaining to soccer injuries. The reasoning behind this is that each sport has its specific requirements concerning fitness, techniques, tactics, team management, and the prevention and treatment of injuries. These conditions required of the soccer player are different from those required of other athletes, such as those who participate in baseball, football, basketball, swimming, etc. There are many volumes written on the care and prevention of athletic injuries, especially to the more popular American sports.

Many authorities feel that whatever the sport, the prevention and treatment of athletic injuries should be the same. At times, this may be a valid statement, but, more commonly, there are slight differences in the best method of treatment for similar injuries. As a soccer player for the past twenty years and a physical therapist for the past sixteen years, the author of this book has had a unique opportunity to experience and care for a wide variety of injuries and can very definitely state the necessity of a different approach in the care and prevention of soccer injuries. The sophistication of the many aspects of the sport, including passing, shooting, and dribbling, in addition to the agility required for running, jumping, etc., necessitates a different approach to injury treatment. Some of the factors to be considered when treating soccer injuries that are different when treating other sports injuries are time for recovery, immediate postinjury exercises, and stretching and strengthening exercises to be done after the acute stage has subsided. Other therapeutic measures, such as applications of heat, cold, water, and electricity, are also used differently.

This book will not contain facts and figures categorizing the differences of treatment in the prevention and correction of similar injuries in different sports. It will proceed with a brief and basic review of the anatomies most involved in soccer injuries. Step-by-step procedures will then be carefully and completely outlined. Hopefully, it will emphasize the need for such a manual on such a subject and will serve two basic functions: (1) to provide an understanding of soccer injuries and (2) to establish an immediate available source of information for coaches, trainers, and soccer players.

The organization of this book poses several problems. What aspects are too irrelevant to include? What information must be included to thoroughly cover the subject? In what order should the basic subjects and methods be placed? Perhaps the reader will not agree with the author's choice, placement, or emphasis. This is a small minus if he finds useful information within these covers.

The author took the liberty in organizing the chapters by first dealing with the treatment and prevention of those soccer injuries that occur most frequently and then the care and prevention of those that occur less frequently. The author has been involved in treating soccer injuries for the past sixteen years.

The most "popular" injuries in soccer are injuries of the lower extremities and specifically those that involve the knee joint. Approximately 50 percent of all the injuries that I have treated involved the knee joint. The next in progression were ankle injuries, thigh injuries, lower leg, lower back, toes, shoulder, abdomen, head and face, respectively. Reviewing the recent N.A.S.L. literature of the past four years regarding the occurrence of soccer injuries, I found considerable similarities as far as their distribution. I will, therefore, proceed in this aforementioned order, devoting a chapter to each. Upon completion of the chapters discussing the care of soccer injuries, I will proceed with a general discussion of conditioning exercises and methods of stretching and strengthening for preseason, during, and after the soccer season. Finally, I would like to emphasize very strongly that a physically fit athlete becomes resistant to most injuries. However, when injuries do occur, I hope this book will be of assistance to the coach, to the trainer, and most of all, to the soccer players.

SOCCER INJURIES:

A Physical Therapy View in Care and Prevention

PART I
GENERAL PHYSICAL THERAPY CONSIDERATIONS

GENERAL DISCUSSION

Physical Therapy is a branch of physical medicine and rehabilitation. It is the branch of physical medicine that employs physical agents such as light, heat, water, and electricity as well as therapeutic exercise for the care and management of injury and/or disease. There are innumerable ways by which the above agents can be applied in the field of soccer injuries or in the field of athletics. In view of the great variety of soccer injuries, the administering of any modality designed for their care should be fully understood before its application. The physical therapist should be able, once a diagnosis has been ascertained, to devise a simple but effective exercise program in great detail of exercise techniques. The physical therapist should be able by using simple terminology to bring a message across to the injured athlete, in effect, not only to reeducate the injured part but to educate the athlete as well.

1. Modalities and Their Application

In the pages to follow, I will briefly enumerate the types of modalities used in physical therapy for the care and prevention of soccer injuries. The application of each modality will be mentioned briefly as well as its mechanics and aftereffects. In doing so, I am hoping to bring into light available information to be used in its practical application. Much of the information included below hasn't been made available before and will further assist the player, the coach, and the trainer in managing soccer injuries.

There are many modalities that are used for the care and prevention of injuries. I will not discuss any sophisticated modalities at this point. I will, however, proceed to discuss their combined efforts, which, when properly applied, provide therapeutic results. The four major derivatives of these modalities are: heat, light, water, and electricity.

Heat

Heat, in physical therapy, is used because it provides local analgesic action. This local action accelerates the process of repair of injured tissues by increasing the local circulation, which is very beneficial for the nutrition of the tissues. When heat is applied in muscular or musculoskeletal disorders after the initial stage, it has the capacity to: (1) relieve pain and discomfort, (2) decrease local spasm and tenderness, and (3) release muscle tightness of muscles and other structures by increasing the mobility of the involved structures. Heat is applied in many forms and through many modalities. I will proceed to list the ones that are most popular as well as fairly simple in their application.

Hydrocollator Hot Packs (Figure 1)

This form of heat is moist and provides warmth to an area by the

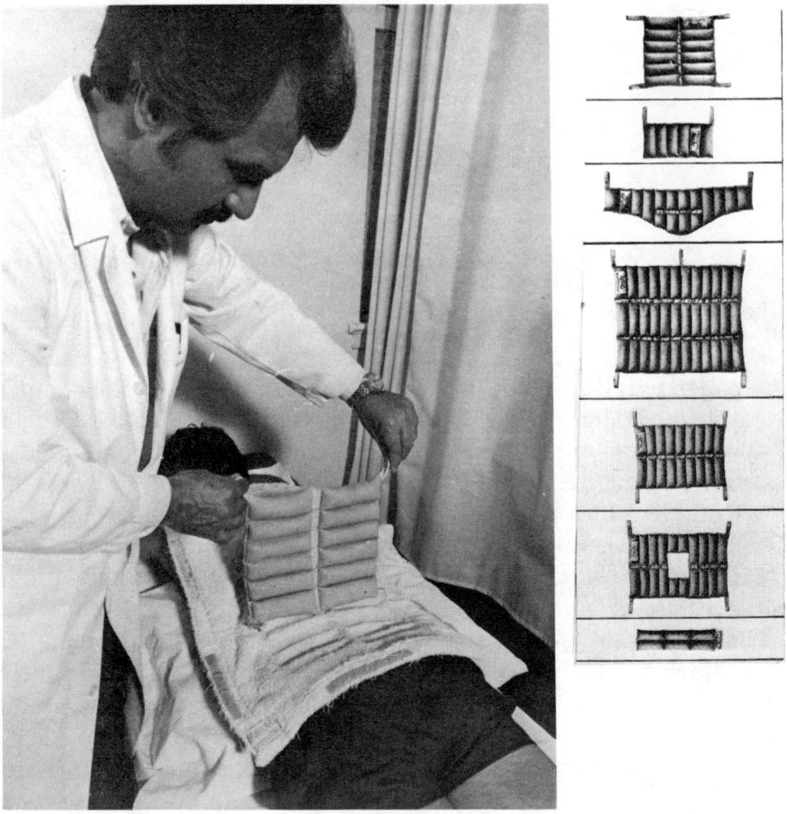

Figure 1. a) Application of hydrocollator hot packs to low back. b) A special cover to insure safety from burning the skin. Different sizes of hot packs for different parts of the body (Courtesy from Geremi Surgicals)

use of chemical pack (salicylate gel) that is preheated in a temperature-controlled tank to the approximate temperature of 135° F. This form of heat is applied to the injured area after it has been insulated with six or eight layers of toweling. Its application lasts between twenty and thirty minutes. Its application usually precedes massage and/or exercise. It is safe, quite effective, and can be operated at a very low cost. It can be used in sprains, strains, and contusions. The nature of hydrocollator heat is superficial.

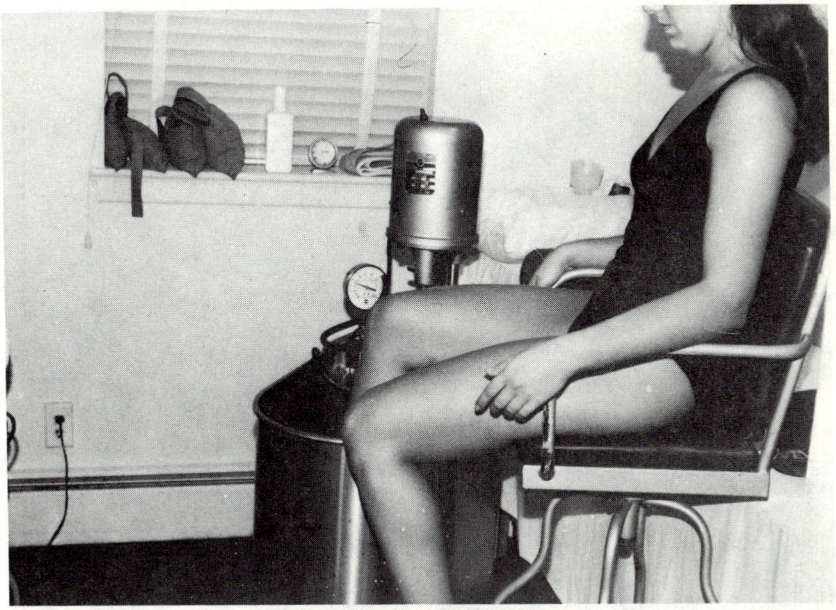

Figure 2. Whirlpool illustrating the motor and the thermometer for keeping desirable water temperature.

Whirlpool (Figure 2)

This form of heat is also moist and superficial in nature. It is very effective because it provides a combination of moisture and heat at the same time. In addition, the water agitator provides gentle massage and muscle relaxation and permits active or assistive exercise of the immersed limb. The duration of the treatment is about 20 minutes, and the water temperature is between 100° and 106° F. Whirlpool treatment is a very simple method of heat application, and its operation is very easy. It is very popular and found in many training rooms.

Diathermy (Short Wave) (Figures 3 and 4)

This is a high-frequency apparatus. It provides heat to the deeper tissues as well as to the more superficial ones. Its application is restricted to a professional who has enough knowledge of the potential dangerous effects of short-wave diathermy. This form of heat is used

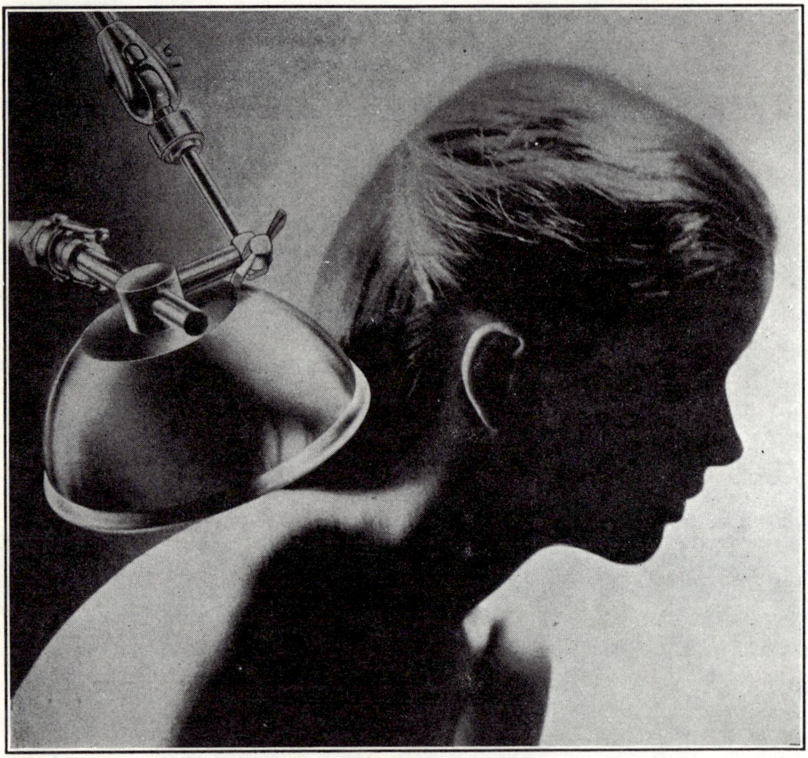

Figure 3. Medical Diathermy—microwave application to shoulder

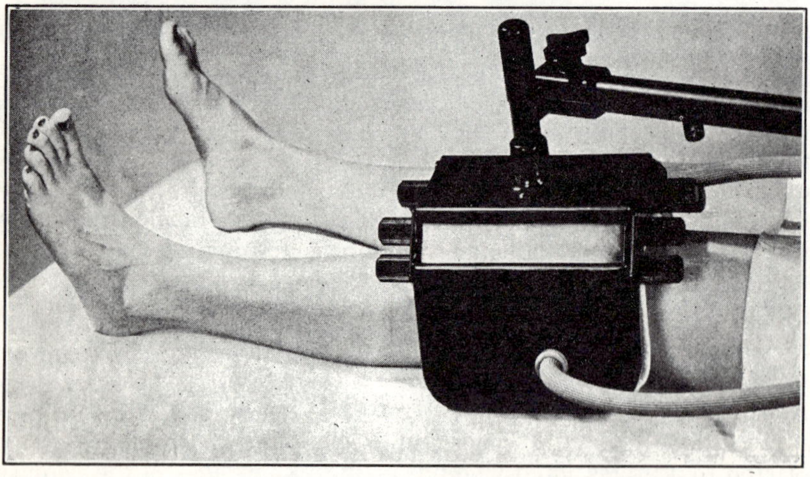

Figure 4. Treatment of knee by hinged electrobe. (Courtesy of the Burdick Corp.)

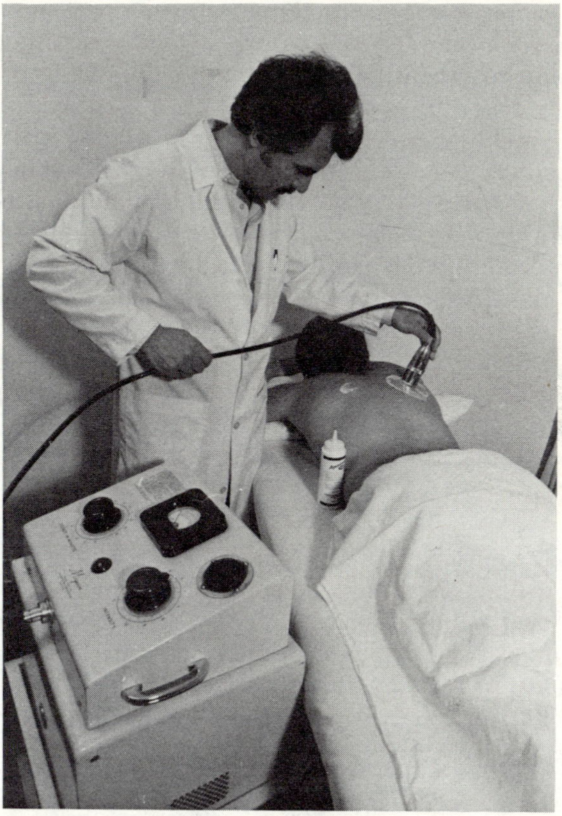

Figure 5. Application of ultrasound showing the applicator and the coupling agent (cream).

very rarely for the management of soccer injuries. In my experience in the care of injuries, short-wave diathermy has been very useful when deep structural damage is involved. Among other contraindications of short-wave diathermy is the presence of imbedded metal. However, in the experience of many observers treating servicemen with shell fragments, screws, or vitallium implants, tissue destruction attributable to the use of short-wave diathermy has not been reported.

Ultrasound (Figure 5)

Ultrasonic therapy, one of the most recently developed methods of heating deep tissues is the energy produced by sound waves. Its application definitely requires the supervision of a professional. Its dosage varies between 0.5 and 2.0 watts/cc.[2] Ultrasonic therapy has been very popular recently for the treatment of soccer and other athletic injuries. When ultrasound is applied, a considerable amount of discretion should be observed. Generally, the athlete will tell you how much intensity will be tolerable. There are athletes, however, who tolerate destructive amounts of ultrasound stimulation because they feel the more they can tolerate, the faster the healing of the injured tissue. Ultrasonic therapy can be applied with a coupling agent such as mineral oil, albalene cream, glycerin, etc. It can also be used indirectly under water when the direct treatment is intolerable even at its minimum dosage. Ultrasonic therapy is suggested generally in most injuries after the acute stage and will assist in the absorption of calcium deposits.

Infrared (Figures 6 and 7)

Infrared radiation produces a superficial heating effect that is used for the relief of muscle spasm and pain, and the increase of local blood supply. Its use has been suggested for the treatment of subacute and chronic traumatic inflammatory conditions such as sprains, strains, and contusions. In addition, fibrositis, tenosynovitis, bursitis, and various forms of arthritis, arthralgia, and néuralgia are symptomatically relieved.

Cold Applications (Figures 8 and 9)

Cold application is the form of treatment mostly used in the acute stage of injury. The length of time to be applied varies between 20 and 30 minutes. This application is combined with compression and elevation. Since most of the injuries are accompanied by swelling, this method impedes the supply of blood, lowers the metabolism locally, and thus prevents further deterioration. Cold should be applied either by commercially available ice packs (with plastic covering) or by self-made water sponges covered by aluminum foil and placed in the freezer. Cold applications should not be applied in the form of full-immersion cold treatment, such as immersing the injured limb in a bucket of water with ice. This form of cold application is contraindicated since frostbite might result. Cold applications may also be used after the initial stage of injury where muscle spasm persists and all other methods of heat applications have failed. In fact, cold and hot applications,

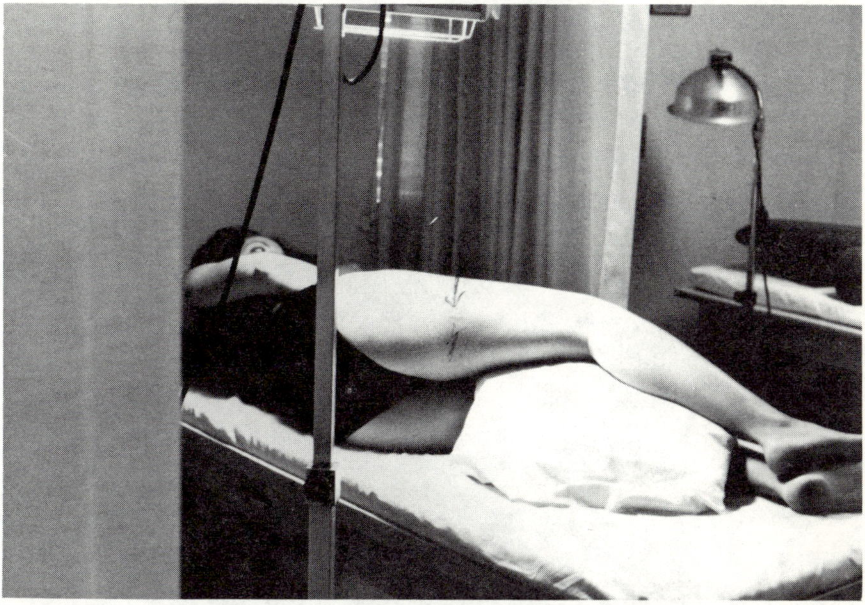

Figure 6. Infrared as applied above injured area. (Courtesy of the Physical Therapy Center of Teaneck, New Jersey)

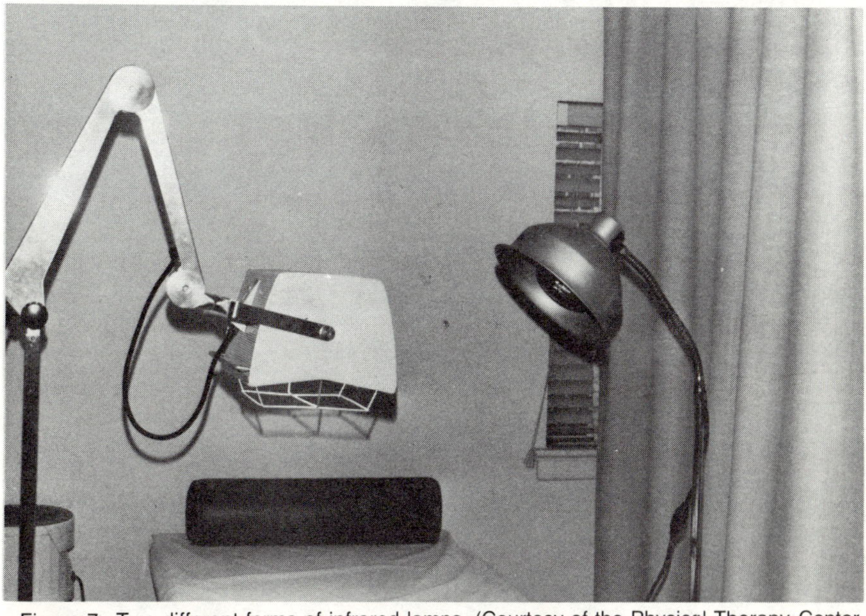

Figure 7. Two different forms of infrared lamps. (Courtesy of the Physical Therapy Center of Teaneck, New Jersey)

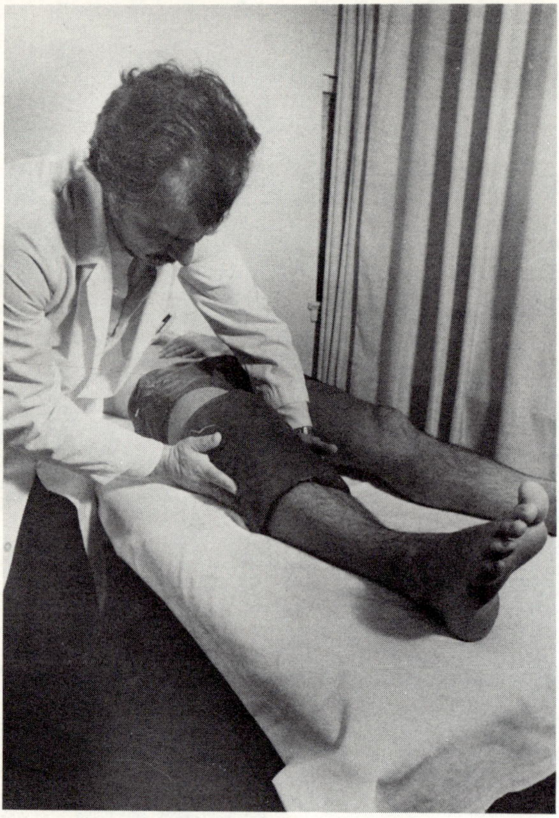

Figure 8 and 9. Hydrocollator ice packs placed over injured knee. They are made from a very pliable substance and fit on the surface easily.

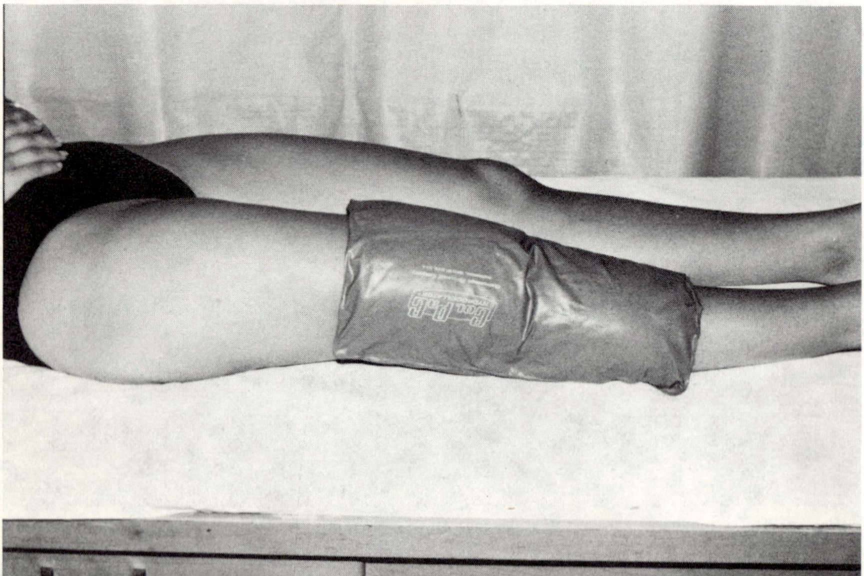

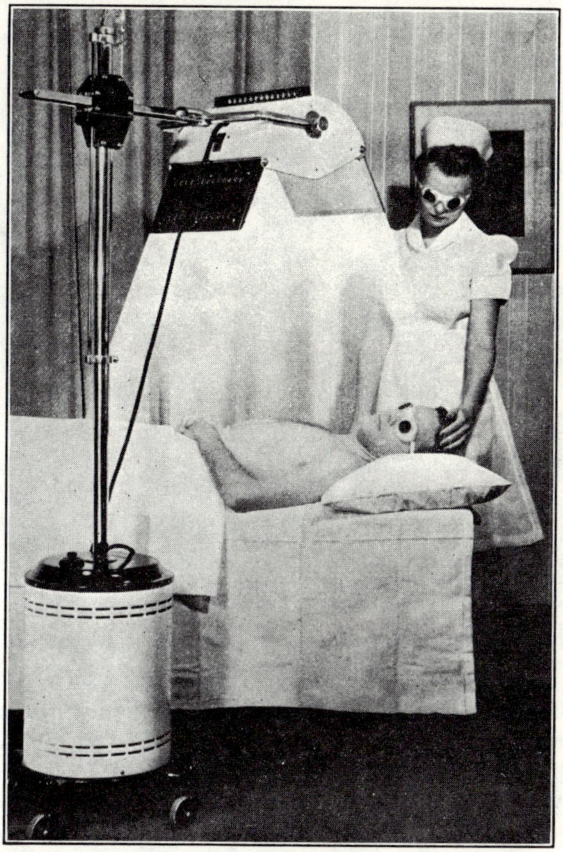

Figure 10. Ultra-violet lamp. (Courtesy of Hanovia Co.)

when used alternately, result in producing relief from pain due to stiffness and the elimination of muscle spasm. In short, when heat and cold are applied alternately to a joint, the treatment prepares the joint for an active exercise program to follow.

Ultraviolet (Figure 10)

Ultraviolet irradiation is seldom being used in soccer injuries. It is mostly indicated for pathological conditions of the skin and other conditions caused by prolonged bed rest known as decubitus ulcers. In athletics, it is being mostly used in conditions of the groin where

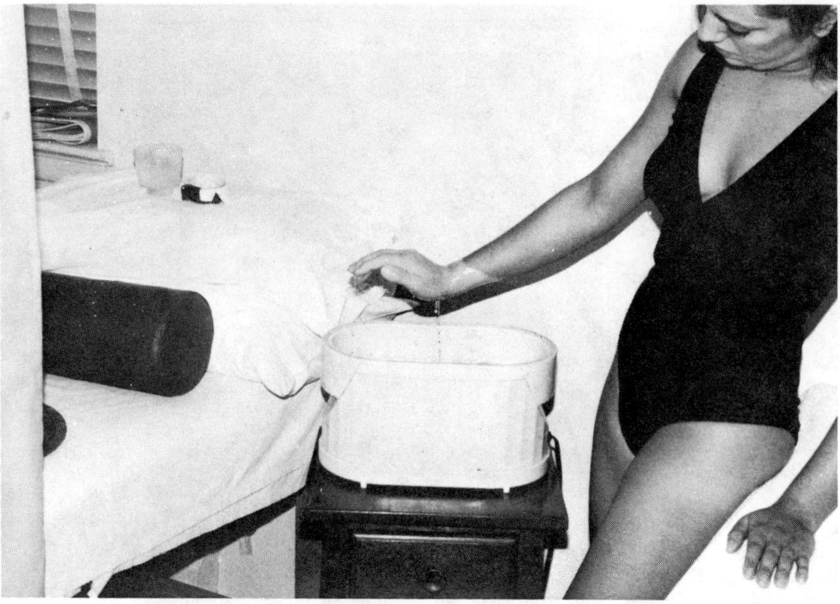

Figure 11. Injured extremity is inserted inside the paraffin several times.

excessive sweat and itching result in infection. Sanitary care combined with ultraviolet will eliminate the infection. The application of ultraviolet should be done strictly by a professional such as a physical therapist who is competent to diagnose its indications and contraindications as well as competent to administer the treatment.

Paraffin Baths (Figure 11)

This form of heat is accomplished by melted wax heated in special tanks at 113–126° F. (45–52° C.). By dipping the limb and withdrawing it several times, the formation of several layers of wax occurs. The limb is then wrapped with grease-proof paper and a towel for 20 to 30 minutes. The heating effect provides relief from pain and is useful to mobilize stiff joints after an injury.

Massage (Figures 12, 13, 14)

"Massage is a systematic and scientific manipulation of the soft tissues of the body." Its stroking has purely French terminology, such

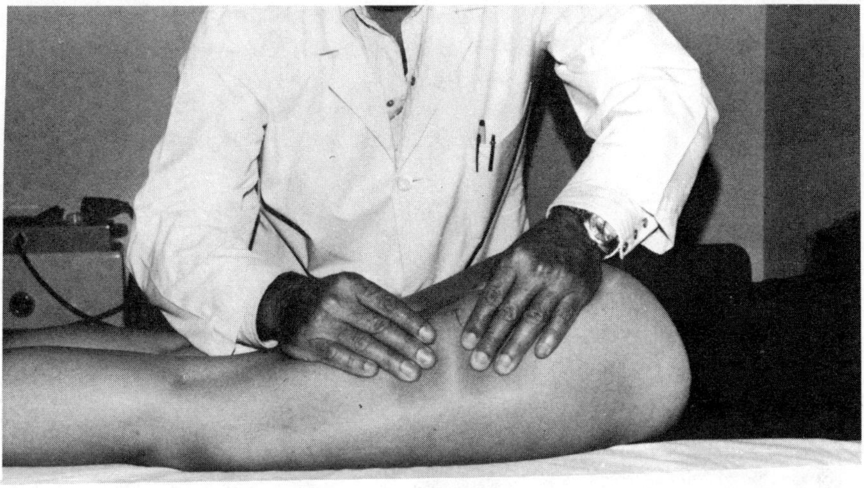

Figure 12. Demonstration of "milking" type of tissue massage.

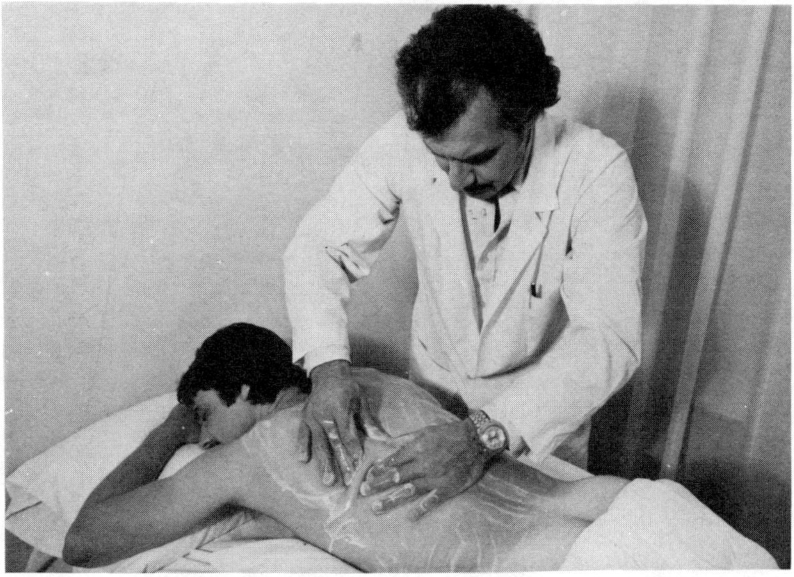

Figure 13. Demonstration of "friction" tissue massage. (Two views)

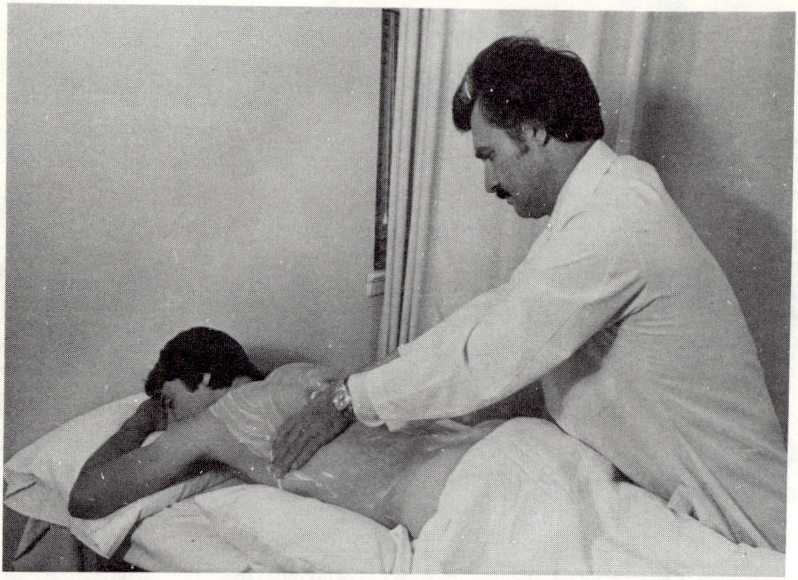

Figure 13. Second View

Figure 14. Demonstration of "knuckling" tissue massage along the spinal column.

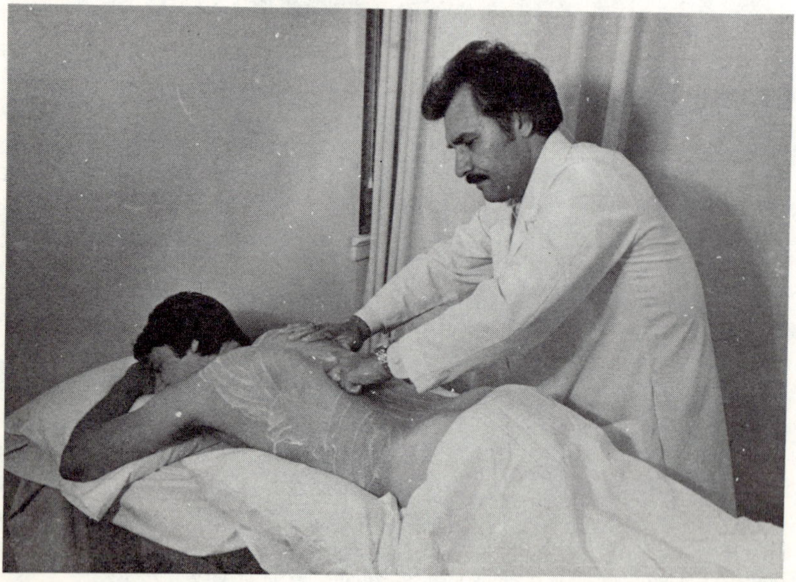

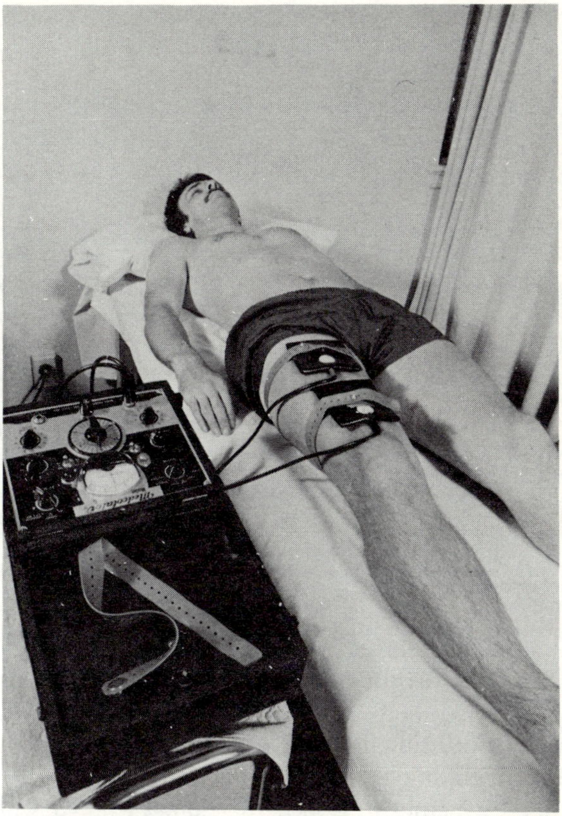

Figure 15. Medcollator, applied along the quadriceps muscles several hours after a pulled muscle.

as: *efflaurage*, meaning gliding; *petrissage,* kneading; *tapotement*, striking; friction, compressing; vibration, vibrating. It is a very ancient method of treatment whose effect fluctuates every decade. Today, massage is indicated in most soccer injuries. Massage can also be used to prepare healthy muscles for strenuous activity or to assist the body to recover from the aftereffects of such activity. The main physiological and psychological effects of massage are: relaxation, relief from pain, reduction of certain types of edema, and increased range of motion.

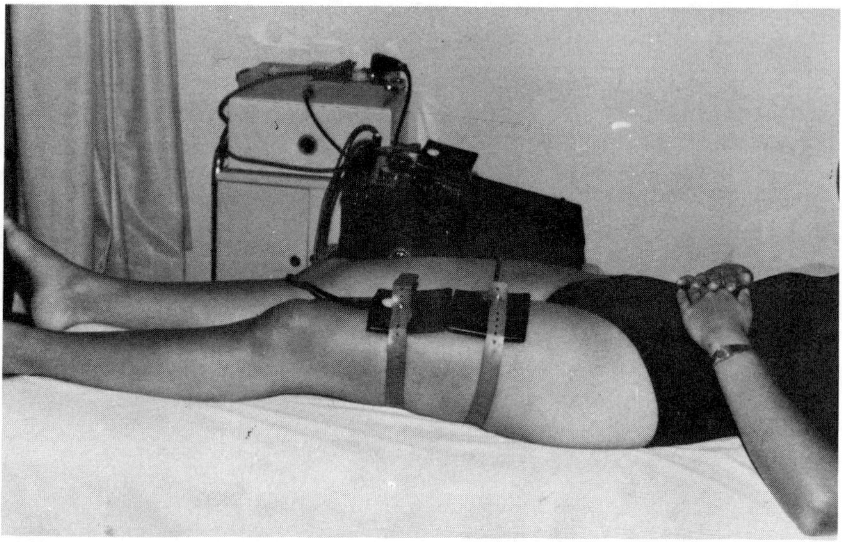

Figure 16. Medcollator.

Electrical Currents (Figures 15, 16, 17)

Electrical stimulation is used extensively in soccer injuries for psychological as well as physical reasons. Psychologically, it gives the athlete a sense of "something is being done" when he observes the involuntary movement of his muscle. Physiologically, we stimulate an injured muscle—in specific situations—in order to retard atrophy from disuse. Although active movement is the best for the restoration of power and function to the muscle, when active movement is not possible, the use of electrical stimulation is suggested. Electrical stimulation is also helpful in improving the circulation and, consequently, the nutrition of the muscle. There are many different modalities that produce electrical stimulation as well as different techniques in applying electrical stimulation. I will briefly name some of the most popular modalities that are being used and found in many physical therapy centers. Some of the most popular electrical stimulation modalities are:

1. Medcollator (Figures 15, 16) provides combination currents of alternating (a.c.) and direct (d.c.), which can be very soothing and very effective.

2. Medcosonlator (Figure 17a) provides the same combination of

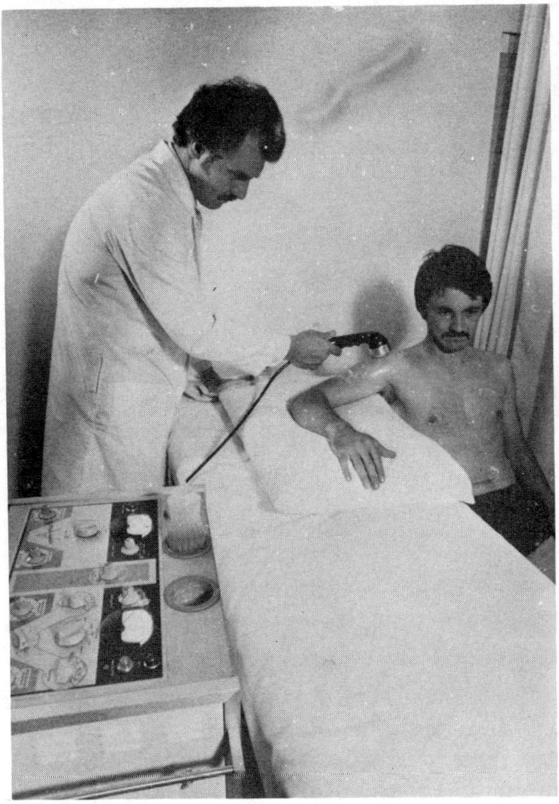

Figure 17a. Medcosonlator, combination of ultra-sound and electrical stimulation.

currents, plus it incorporates and utilizes ultrasound along with the stimulation, which, when combined, soothes the painful trigger points of the injured area.

3. Transcutaneous electrical nerve stimulation, the most recent form of pain-relieving agent, whose stimulating, soothing effect is still under clinical investigation. For the limited time that I have been involved with it, I believe it has potential use as an adjunct to other therapeutics for the care and prevention of soccer injuries. (Figure 17b)

General Comments

All of the above modalities that I have discussed most definitely

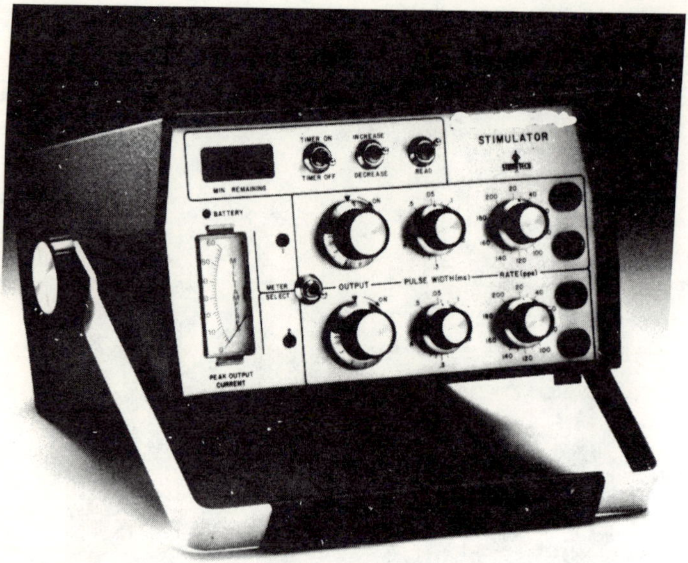

Figure 17b. Transcutaneous electrical nerve stimulation.

require the active participation or supervision of a professional such as a physical therapist. Every modality has advantages and disadvantages as well as indications and contraindications. For this reason, only a trained person will be able to recognize both and apply the proper technique and/or the proper dosage for treatment that is indicated and also therapeutically advantageous.

2. Strengthening Techniques

Exercise is an essential aspect of the rehabilitation of muscles that have become weak either directly after an injury and/or after surgery. Usually, weakness results from disuse in both cases. The type of exercise program designed for muscle weakness will depend on the site of the injury, the degree of the injury, and the extent of the muscle involvement. If only a small muscle has been injured, then our concern will be to design a program to strengthen this particular muscle and then incorporate in the same program the surrounding group of muscles. If the involvement is general, then a general exercise program should be designed in which progressive strengthening techniques will be more applicable. A trained physical therapist with proficiency in kinesiology (study of muscle movement) will easily recognize the imbalance of muscle strength and, consequently, will design the proper strengthening program for the involved muscles. Exercises have many physiological effects:

1. Increase circulation
2. Increase muscular strength
3. Increase muscular endurance
4. Assist normal range of motion
5. Prevent atrophy
6. Assist in reestablishing movement

There are four major forms of exercise:

1. Passive exercise
2. Active assistive exercise
3. Active exercise
4. Progressive resistive exercise

Passive Exercise

This form of exercise is very rarely used in athletics. It is mostly used in spinal cord injuries in which there is paralysis of limbs and other neuromuscular involvements. In athletics, stretching is considered to be a part of passive exercise, and it is used mostly before and after strenuous muscular activity. It is used before for preventive measures to avoid muscular injuries such as muscle pulls, strains, and contusions. It is used after strenuous activity for relaxation purposes and for the impediment of fatigue. Stretching should be done very slowly, maintaining the maximum range for several seconds. Forced movement may result in muscle damage and loss of mobility. Sustained moderate stretching is more effective than instantly vigorous stretching.

Active-Assistive Exercise

This type of exercise is usually designed after a severe sprain or a fracture of an extremity. The athlete is assisted by the therapist to complete the normal range of movement. (For example, in a partial tear of the quadriceps the athlete will be assisted to flex his knee joint while lying on his stomach.) This type of assistance requires professional judgment regarding the amount of force indicated.

Active Exercise

This form of exercise is performed by the athlete himself. Active exercise, being antonomous (functioning independently), incorporates all local parts of the locomotor system and thus encourages full range of motion, strengthens the muscles, and impedes the development of adhesions and, consequently, muscle tightness. Active exercise is advocated after prolonged immobilization, as, for example, after a fracture. This form of exercise can be graded in the number of progressive repetitions, depending on the ability of the athlete.

Progressive Resistive Exercise (P.R.E.)

This type of exercise incorporates a very large part in the rehabilitative program of the injured player. Resistive exercise following soccer injuries is not a new concept for the restoration of muscle strength. De Lorme, in 1945, described a system that, after many revisions, became known as 10 Repetitions Maximum (the maximal resistance the muscle can lift through the full range of motion after

10 repetitions). Determine the 10 repetition maximal resistance, that is, 10 R.M., by contracting the muscle 10 times and progressively increasing the resistance for bouts of 10 contractions each until the maximum resistance that can be lifted 10 times is reached. For each exercise, five days weekly, have the athlete perform 10 bouts of 10 contractions each, beginning at 10 percent of 10 R.M. and proceed to a 100 percent of 10 R.M. by increasing the load daily by 10 percent daily of 10 R.M. This system becomes time consuming, especially when the trainer has to establish the new 10 R.M. for the following week. The newer of P.R.E. by De Lorme demonstrates shortened sequences of progression, which prove to be just as effective in improving muscle strength. Thus,

First set of 10 repetitions—use one half of 10 R.M.

Second Set of 10 repetitions—use three quarters of 10 R.M.

Third Set of 10 repetitions—use full 10 R.M.

This above method of De Lorme's is mostly used for strengthening the quadriceps muscles. To illustrate this method, which is quite time consuming, I will use a hypothetical example, which will be divided into four steps.

Step 1. The athlete is using light weights for warming up his quadriceps (Figure 18). The maximum weight the athlete can lift one time will be 20 pounds.

Step 2. The maximum weight that has been established is divided in half or 10 pounds and is lifted 10 times; Rest for 2 minutes.

Step 3. The maximum weight in step 1 is divided into three quarters or 15 pounds and is lifted 10 times; Rest for 2 minutes.

Step 4. The maximum load or 20 pounds is lifted 10 times.

Note: In treating knee injuries, I have slightly modified this method by eliminating the fourth step, where the athlete should lift the maximum weight of step 1, 10 times. In my experience, the fourth step is never performed satisfactorily, and the athlete becomes discouraged. Furthermore, as you noticed in step 1, I have eliminated the 10 repetitions maximum for the top weight, and instead I used 1 repetition maximum for the top weight. Therefore, the athlete will proceed to base his second and third step from the top weight of step 1.

To illustrate this further mathematically:

Step 1. 1 Repetition Maximum (1 R.M.) = 20 pounds.

Step 2. 1 R.M. = 20 × ½ or 10 pounds lifted 10 times.

Step 3. 1 R.M. = 20 × ¾ or 15 pounds lifted 10 times.

The above three steps repeated three times daily for three days per week. At the end of the week, again we proceed with step 1 to find the maximum weight lifted one time. It is anticipated that the 1 R.M. will be greater than the previous 20 pounds, to perhaps 25 or 30 pounds. In well-trained athletes, it is not necessary to wait until the end of the week before you proceed to find the 1 R.M. This can be done at the end of each treatment session, after the athlete has completed his three sets of the three steps indicated previously.

Equipment

N/K table or a quadriceps table is much more preferable than the traditional iron boot and cross-bar clamps. In fact, for safety purposes, the iron boot and weights at the ankle would be totally eliminated because the direct downward force that is applied at the knee joint has a tendency to stretch the collateral ligaments and the menisci. This can be easily eliminated by not permitting the knee to start extension from 90° but from 110°; this way, the downward force is eliminated. However, even starting at 110°, isokinetically, is not indicated because the desirable resistance is not applied throughout the entire range. I would, therefore, recommend the use of a quadriceps exercise table with levers and/or hydraulic pressure for easier access to the desirable amount of resistance, and at the same time eliminate the chances of stretching the knee ligaments. (Figure 18e)

Assuming that such a table is available, the athlete positions himself or herself (more and more women are involved with soccer) at the end of the table with a small pillow or a rolled towel under the thigh proximal to the knee joint. The leg hangs over the table and the athlete begins to extend his leg to full extension against the predetermined resistive force. Once the full extension has been reached, it must be maintained for six seconds or a slow count of six. The player's hands are placed either on his chest or behind, grasping the table for maintaining his balance. If the full extension can not be reached, then obviously the weight is too heavy and should be changed to a lighter one.

Other methods similar to De Lorme's can be used for strengthening exercises, such as McGovern and Luscombe, who advocated a reversal of the 10 R.M., which means using the full 10 R.M. in the first set and one-half in the third set. One other method that I have been using in addition to De Lorme's and that is preferred by many athletes because of its repetitions is the one that I call two-thirds of 1 R.M. times 30 repetitions. It implies that once the 1 R.M. is found, subtract one third of the top load and ask the athlete to lift 30 times in groups of 10, with 1 minute rest between groups. During this minute, the athlete who is

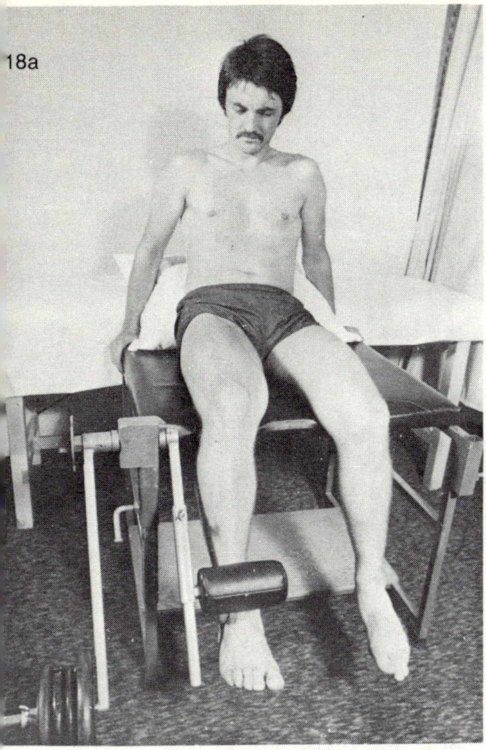

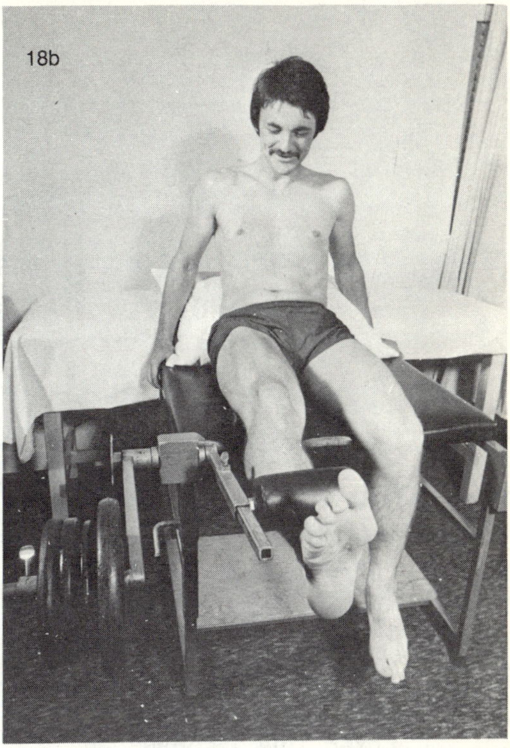

Figure 18. Applying the P.R.E. technique on the N/K (quadriceps table). Steps a) and b) for the quadriceps; c) and d) for the hamstrings.

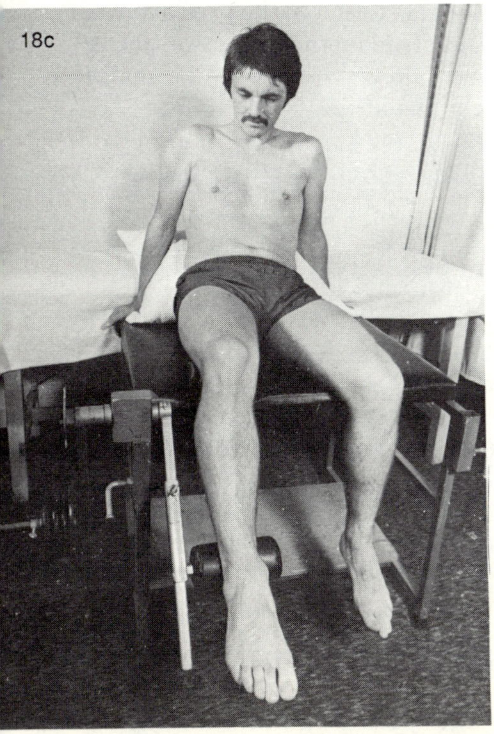

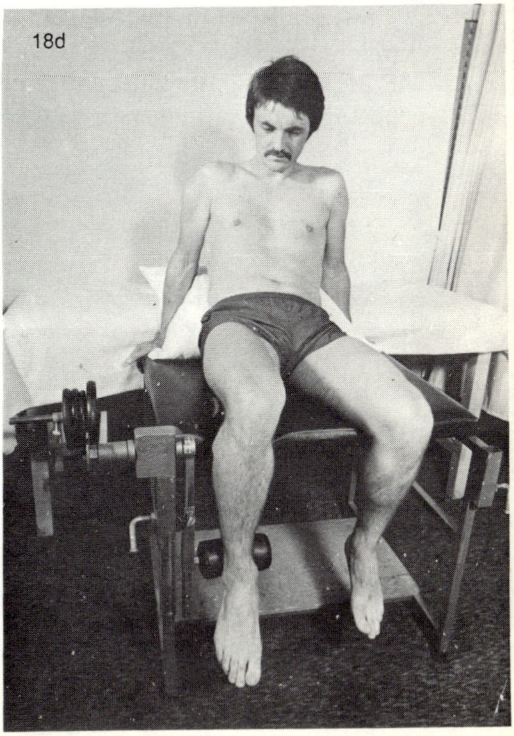

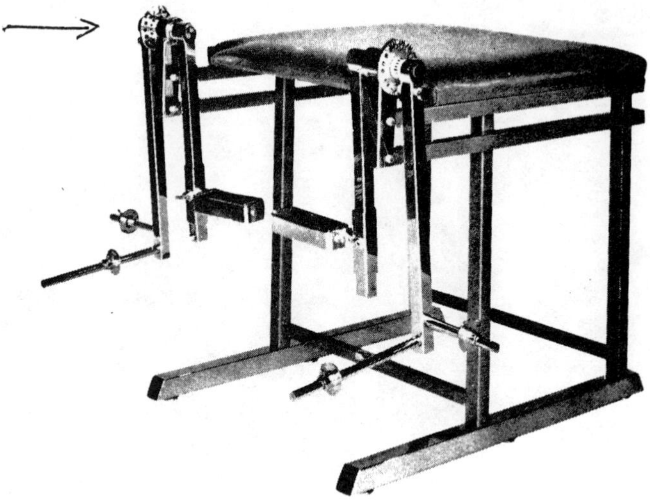

Figure 18e. N/K Table (Courtesy of Geremi Surgicals Inc.)

is exercising his quads, now is reversing his force and presses down, thus resisting his hamstrings or flexing his knee. When the minute is up, he continues his completion of 30 repetitions. The physiological advantage of using the opposite muscles (antagonists), in this case, the hamstrings, while resting is to provide relaxation to the prime movers (agonists), in this case, the quadriceps. This method, the two-thirds 1 R.M. times 30, has been very effective along with the De Lorme's in postoperative and/or postinjury care of the knee.

3. Bandaging Techniques

The immediate treatment after an injury is aimed to minimize the hemorrhage (any discharge of blood from the blood vessels caused by injury) and the hematoma (a circumscribed collection of blood following trauma) and to shorten the period of convalescence. In acute sprains, strains, and contusions, the treatment should include cold packs and compression bandage, both applied to reduce the accumulation of clot formation and, consequently, the amount of scar laid down in the tissues. Bandaging is defined as "the art of applying adaptable material to the limbs or body for the purpose of control." In discussing bandaging techniques, we are involved in a wide variety of both kinds of bandages, and methods of bandaging. We will, however, proceed to discuss those kinds and methods that are more prevalent in soccer injuries and those that I think are practical and effective in their application.

Note: Whatever bandage is decided to be used, the method of its application must be regulated by certain rules: (1) to allow muscle contraction; (2) to allow free flow of blood (not to restrict circulation); (3) it should start from the distal and move to the proximal covering the injured part; (4) the part to be bandaged should be placed in a functional position; (5) it should follow the contours of the injured limb and must stay flat, (6) when applicable, to hold the dressings or splints in position; (7) to limit movement; and (8) to protect and support the injured area. The most practical and effective technique in bandaging is the figure eight. It is practical because it is easily applicable in any extremity. It is effective because its form does not restrict the blood flow but assists the flow from distal to proximal in a uniform capacity. The figure eight is being used quite effectively in ankle and knee injuries as well as in wrist and elbow injuries. Figure-eight bandaging can also be applied in injuries of mid and upper thigh, with the bandage anchored along the waist in front of the abdominal wall. For abdominal bandaging figure eight, it can be applied with the loops crossing over in the front of the abdominal wall. (Figures 19, 20, 21a, b, c, d, e).

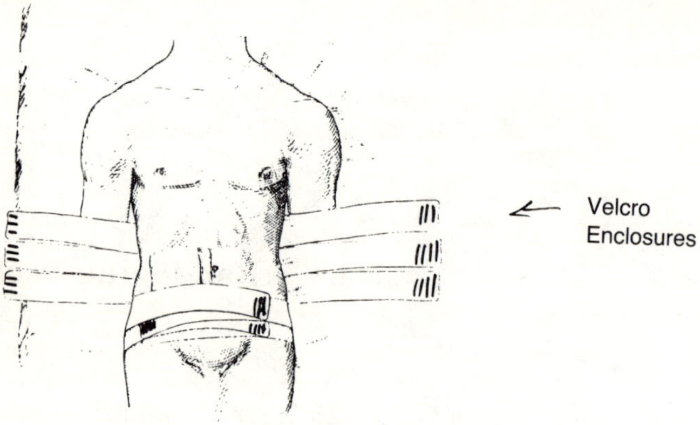

Figure 19. Abdominal bandaging—arrow pointing sponge at painful area.

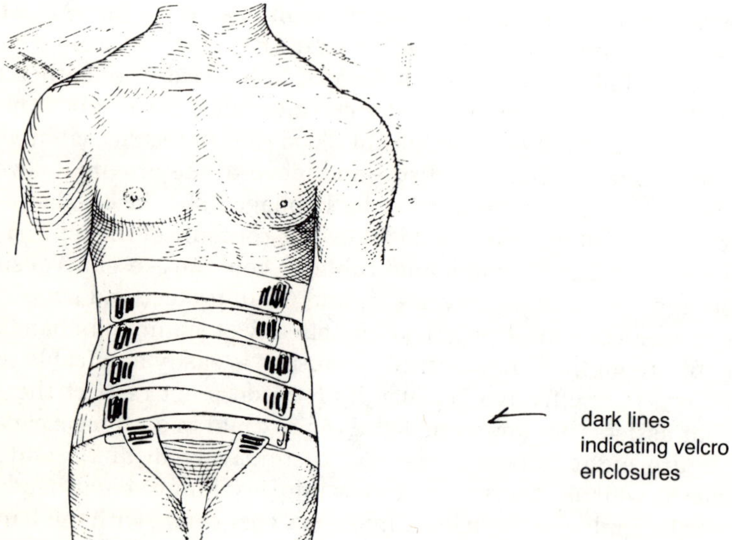

Figure 20. Abdominal bandaging, complete (observe velcro enclosures).

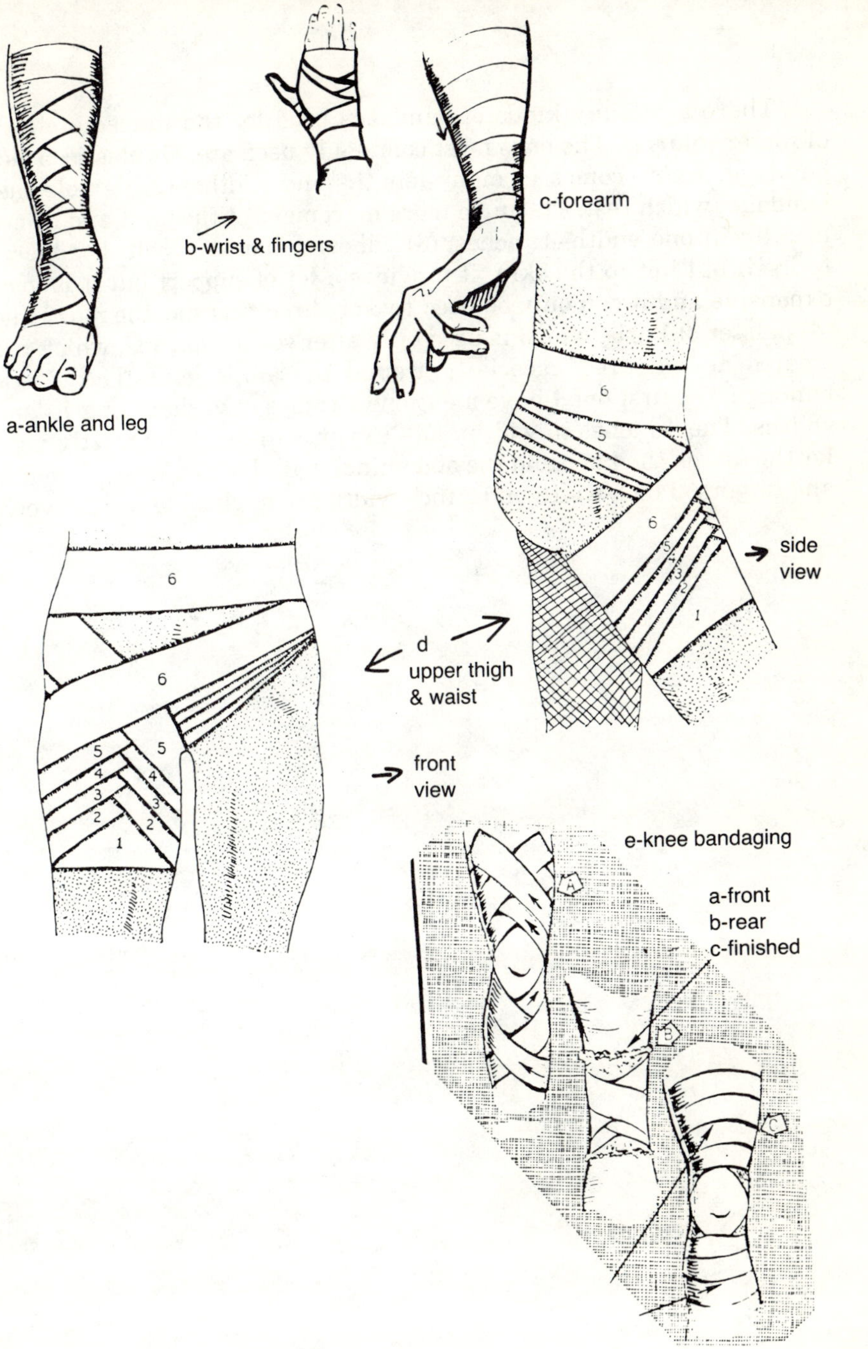

Figure 21. Figure-eight bandaging a) ankle and leg, b) wrist and finger, c) forearm, d) upper thigh and waist, e) knee bandaging. front view, side view

There are many kinds of bandages used for the immediate care of soccer injuries. The ones most commonly used are: (1) elastic or ace bandage, which comes in many lengths and widths; (2) flexible cast bandage, which restricts much more movement at the joint and comes usually in one width–4 inches; (3) adhesive bandage, which adheres to itself but not to the skin; it provides a lot of support but it is very expensive and it can only be used two or three times at the most; and (4) plaster of Paris, which is used only after severe sprains, which are treated as fractures, especially around the ankle joint. The elastic bandage, the first one I have mentioned, comes in various lengths and widths. The 4 inches in width and 2½ yards in length is mostly used for the ankle, the knee and the abdominal wall. For the wrist, forearm and fingers, 3 inch width and 2 inch width are applicable respectively.

4. Taping Techniques

The principle of applying tape in soccer injuries is very important primarily to prevent deterioration of previous injury rather than as a normal procedure in pregame preparation for American football. In soccer injuries, taping is mostly used in ankle injuries, and it is applicable in postinjury care. Should taping be used on ankles in pregame preparation, the player's performance will be greatly reduced. The primary function of taping is to limit movement wherever it is applied. When movement around the ankle joint is limited, then the performance in the area of technique application is limited as well. Indeed, there are situations in which the participation of a particular player is necessary. Under these conditions, therefore, it is up to the coach, in cooperation with the trainer, to see that a good taping job is applied with the least possible restrictive movement but with considerable amount of support.

Let me point out, however, that in view of the sophistication of the game of soccer and its multiplicity of interchangeable movements such as passing, shooting, and dribbling, it is quite impossible to find taping techniques that will permit all of the above and yet provide support at the same time. I would, therefore, suggest taping to be used for postinjury care for sprains, strains, etc., for full or partial immobilization, to alleviate discomfort and encourage rapid healing.

A considerable knowledge of the anatomical structures of the extremities involved is very important so that the application of the tape will be of value. The improper application of taping not only will cause pain and discomfort, but it will impede the process of healing as well. Its primary function, therefore, should be to permit faster healing by bringing injured parts closer together, thus promoting repair.

General rules in preparation for taping

1. Clean the area to be taped.

2. Any laceration or abrasion must be covered before the application of the tape.

3. Shave the area before taping—now it is not absolutely necessary in view of the existing pretape self-adhesive material that is commercially available.

4. Position the part to be taped in the proper anatomic position (see ankle taping, Figures 22, 23).

5. Select the proper size of adhesive tape usually 1″ or 2″ in width, the most commonly used adhesive tape.

6. Do not allow the tape to wrinkle.

7. When taping the ankle, the application of small gauzes at the front of the ankle and at the heel cord will prevent irritations.

8. Apply tape firmly but avoid circular movements, which will constrict circulation.

9. Each strip of tape must overlap the preceding to avoid exposed skin and eventual skin irritation.

10. If pain and discomfort are experienced immediately after the application of tape, the taping has been applied incorrectly. Remove it and reapply it.

11. When removing tape, exercise as much care as when it was applied.

12. Do not remove by tearing, ripping, or pulling.

13. Remove tape by applying vertical and horizontal cuts with special safety adhesive scissors.

14. If tape has been applied directly to the skin—preferably with the use of pretape material—use spray remover and cleanse the area with alcohol, followed by powder or calamine lotion.

15. Avoid the use of taping after whirlpool baths, hot pack applications, or other heat modalities in which heat is discharged from the skin. If taping is necessary, the area to be applied must be dry.

For further demonstrations of taping techniques, see Figures 25a, 25b, 26, 27, 28.

The most common application of taping for ankle support is known as the Gibney application, probably after the man who first applied it. There are six main steps of an open-faced Gibney.

Step 1: Start the tape approximately above the medial malleolus (ankle bone); pull the tape around the heel, close and parallel to the tendon of Achilles. The tape will end about 6 inches above the lateral malleolus (ankle bone outside of leg). Press tape down with the palm of the hand.

Step 2: Start at the base of the great toe, pull the tape around the heel, and run it parallel with the bottom of the foot and as close as

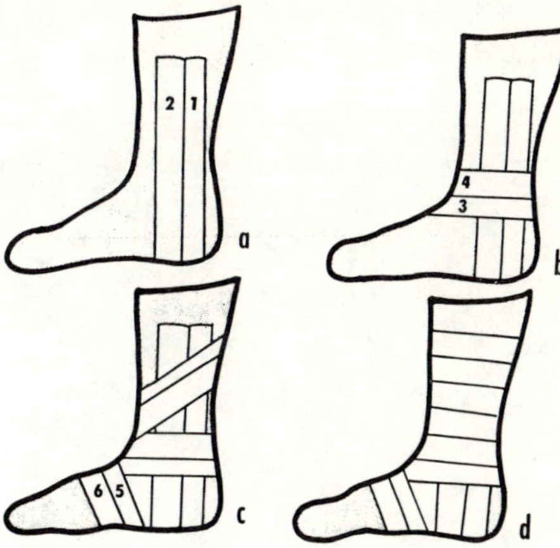

Figure 22. Regular strapping using vertical and horizontal strips.

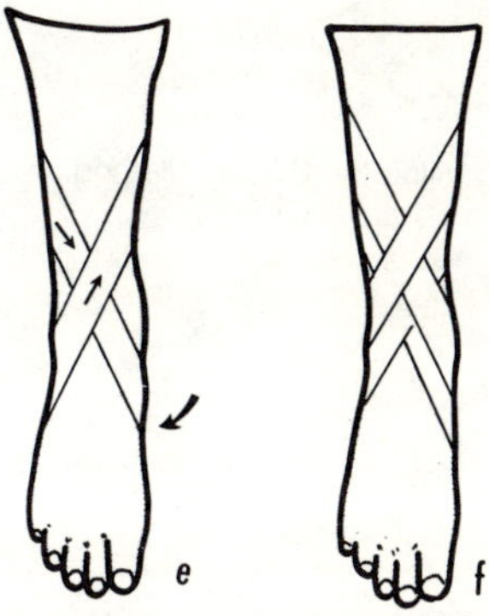

Figure 23. Ankle strapping using diagonal strips, bringing the foot gradually to a neutral position.

possible to the sole. Finish at the base of the little toe.

Step 3: Repeat step 1, overlapping at least halfway.

Step 4: Repeat step 2, starting about one quarter inch short of strip two and overlapping at least halfway.

Step 5: Repeat step 1; usually, three to four vertical strips will be adequate.

Step 6: Repeat the horizontal strips all the way up to the start of the vertical strips. Recess each one so that the front of the foot and ankle remains visible. Another type of ankle taping is known as ankle strap with figure eight, which is essentially the Gibney with variations

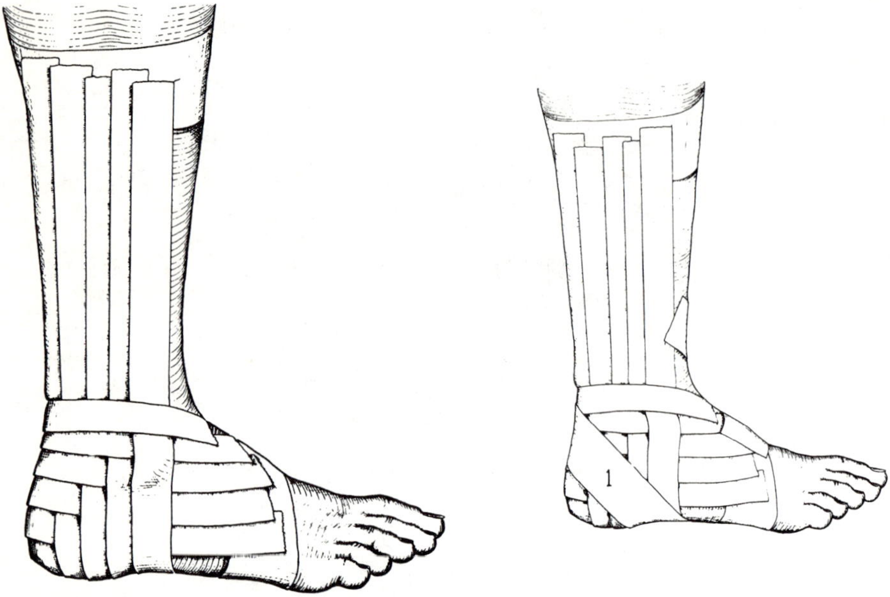

Figure 24a, b. Ankle strapping using the Gibney Method.

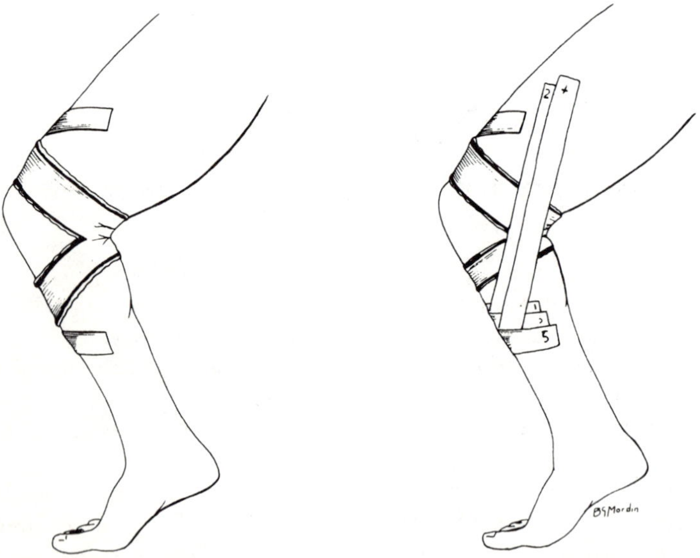

Figure 25a, b. Duke Simpson strapping, for prevention of recurrent sprains of the knee.

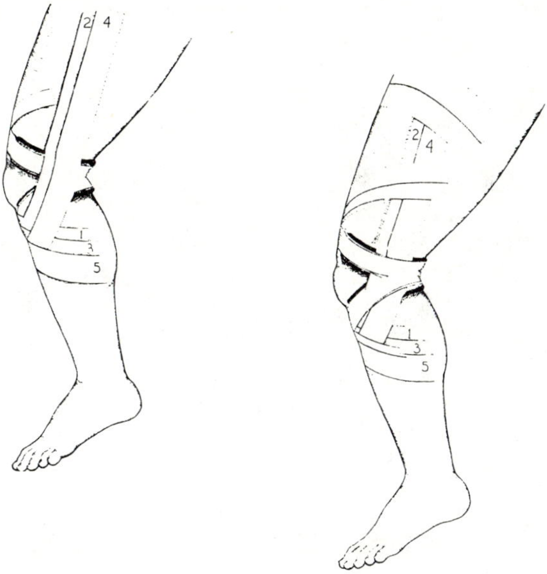

Figure 26. Taping and splinting of the knee.

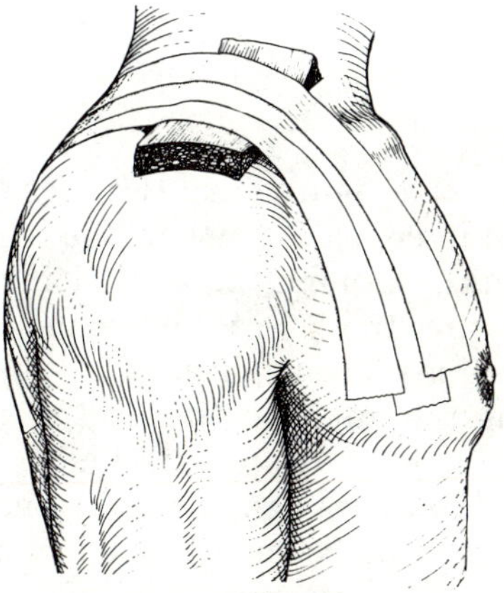

Figure 27. Taping for acromioclavicular sprains using a felt pad.

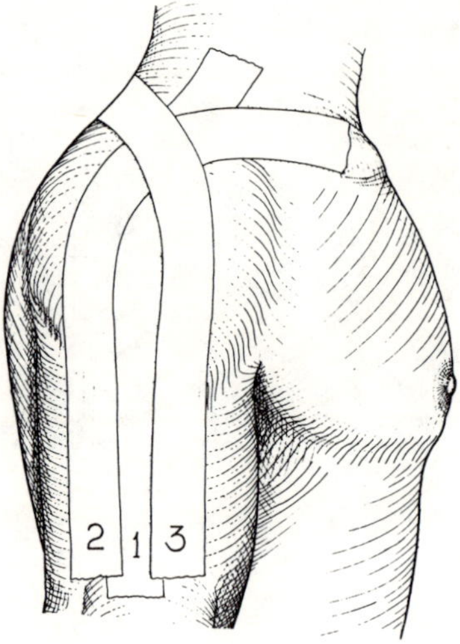

Figure 28. Taping for deltoid contusions and/or acromioclavicular sprains.

and a reinforcement with a figure eight (Figures 24a, b).

I have attempted to describe a few methods, with many illustrations, of taping primarily around the ankle joint. In view of the mechanics of the ankle joint, the lateral ligaments are injured ten times more than the medial ones. The application of taping, however, should be the same, keeping the ankle in the neutral position. I have not attempted to describe any knee-taping techniques because I felt that the illustrations would be clear enough. Furthermore, specific knee injuries and their care will be mentioned in later chapters. Other taping techniques with illustrations of different areas of the body are also available. (Figures 29a, 29b, 29c, 29d, 29e).

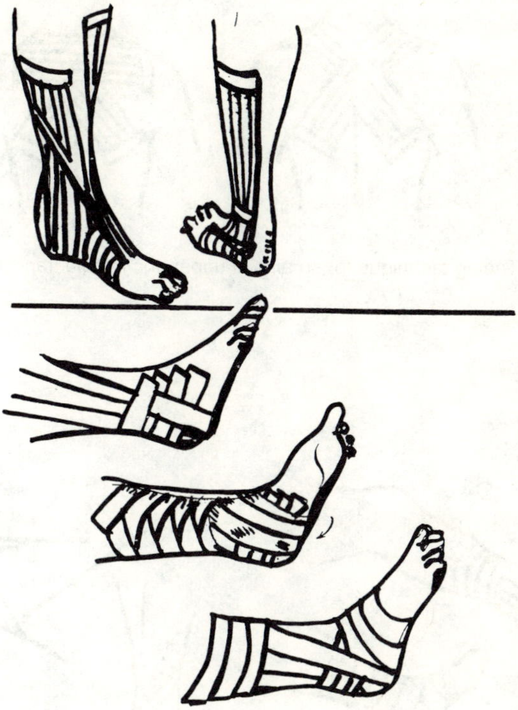

Figure 29a. Ankle strapping with flexible casting strips.

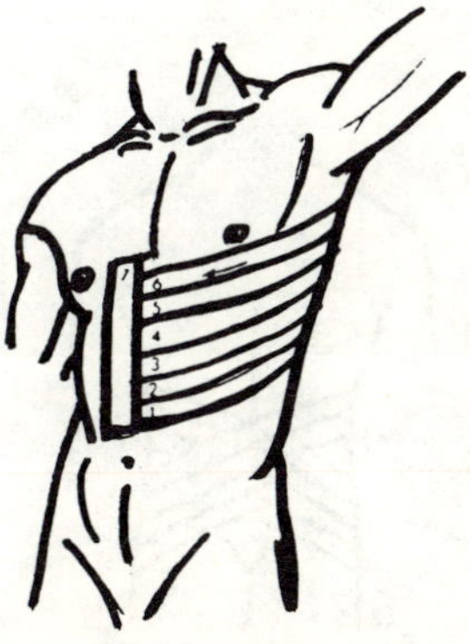

Figure 29b. Taping techniques for sprains of the serratus anterior, as well as rib strain.

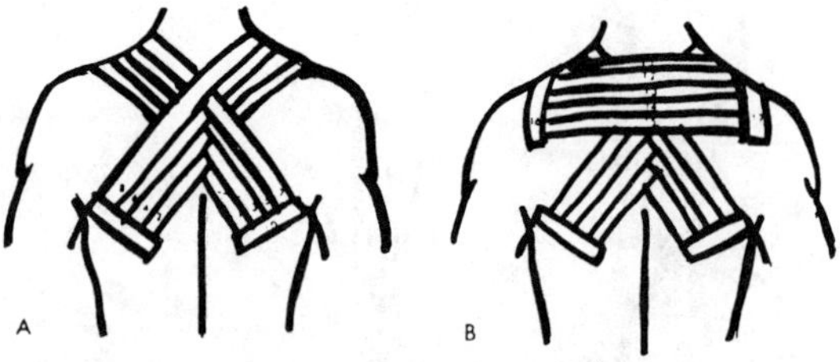

Figure 29c. Taping technique for sprains of upper and middle trapezius.

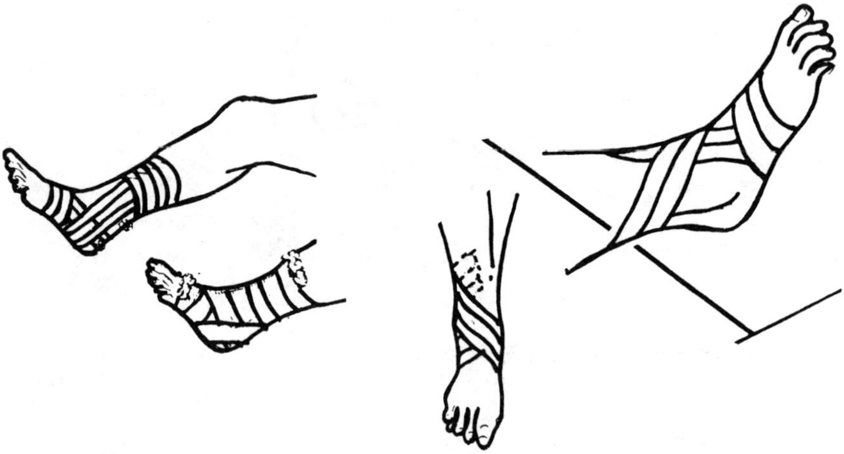

Figure 29d. Other methods of ankle strapping with flexible casting strips.

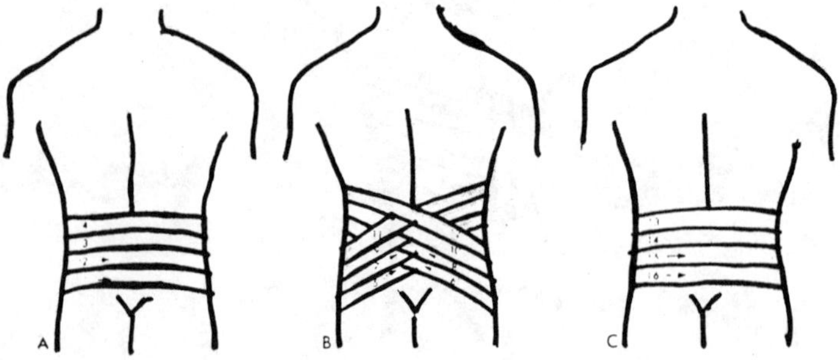

Figure 29e. Taping for low back strain; three separate layers of tape.

5. Ethyl Chloride Application Technique

The application of ethyl chloride in soccer injuries should not be overemphasized and labeled as the chosen treatment immediately after injury. We have often seen enough trainers who run in the middle of the field when an injury occurs with a spray can of ethyl chloride in their hands. The use of ethyl chloride spray is only effective in eliminating painful muscle spasm that results from local injury. When ethyl chloride spray is used to reduce muscle swelling through its chilling effect, it is not only misused but could result in causing various degrees of burn. Ethyl chloride spray can be used as a local anaesthetic agent to render temporary relief in such conditions as muscle contusions and joint or muscle sprains that are painful and cause restriction of movement, provided there is no fracture, torn muscles, or ligamentous tear.

Ethyl chloride, when applied as above indicated, has the following advantages:

1. Assists restoration of normal function.
2. Shortens treatment time (prevention better than correction).
3. Relieves muscle spasm.
4. Prevents joint stiffness.
5. Impedes swelling.
6. Cuts down recovery time.
7. Eliminates extensive treatment.
8. Puts the player back in the game faster.
9. It can be used as a diagnostic tool as follows: (1) if complete relief is derived after its application, it would indicate a simple sprain; (2) if there is continuous deep pain after its application, it would indicate serious damage.

Method of Application (Technique)

1. Apply thin layer of petroleum jelly on the area.

2. Spray ethyl chloride from 10 to 18 inches from the target.

3. When skin blanches (approximately 30 seconds), stop spray.

4. Ask athlete to move through the range of the injured part.

5. Ask him to pinpoint exact areas of pain.

6. Spray again until frost appears or he complains of burning sensations.

7. In an ankle injury, have athlete go through the range of motion, first lying down and then standing on his toes.

8. Instruct exercises: (1) dorsi flexion, (2) plantar flexion, (3) inversion, (4) eversion, (5) heel-toe walking, (6) walking naturally.

9. Ask athlete again to pinpoint areas of pain.

10. Reapply for the last time ethyl chloride if pain is mild at the pointed areas.

11. Apply additional therapeutic adjuncts such as whirlpool for 15 minutes at 85–90° F during early stages—first 24 hours. To be followed with 105–110° F after 24 hours.

6. Measurement of Range of Motion (R.O.M.)

There are many complaints expressed by an athlete after an injury—pain, weakness, clumsiness of movement—that are related to movement and, consequently, to motor activity. The lack of motor activity, consequently, is dependent on the range of motion of one or more joints. During the evaluation of a postinjured athlete, the range of motion testing is very important in determining the degree of injury. The range of motion of each joint of the human body has been predetermined by experts, who used such instruments as "arthrometers" (instruments of measuring joints), "goniometers" (instruments for measuring angles), or "fleximeters" (instruments for measuring the degree of bending). The most common instrument used today in physical therapy to measure the range of motion of any peripheral joint is the goniometer. The next best method to estimate and evaluate range of motion limitations is experience. One can learn to estimate fairly accurately the maximal range of motion of a joint. Below, there are illustrative charts pointing out the normal ranges throughout joints

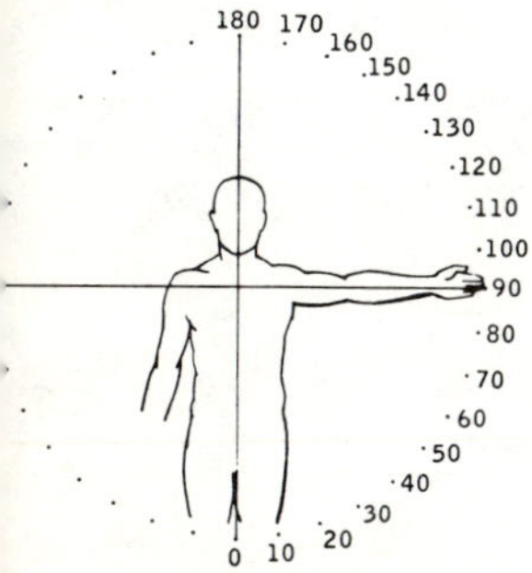

SHOULDER

Abduction	0 – 90
Abd. & Rot. Scapula*	90 – 180
Add. & Rot. Scapula	180 – 90
Adduction	90 – 0

LIMITATIONS

	L		R	
	Abd.	Add.	Abd.	Add.
1				
2				
3				
4				

* Rot.—Rotation of scapula

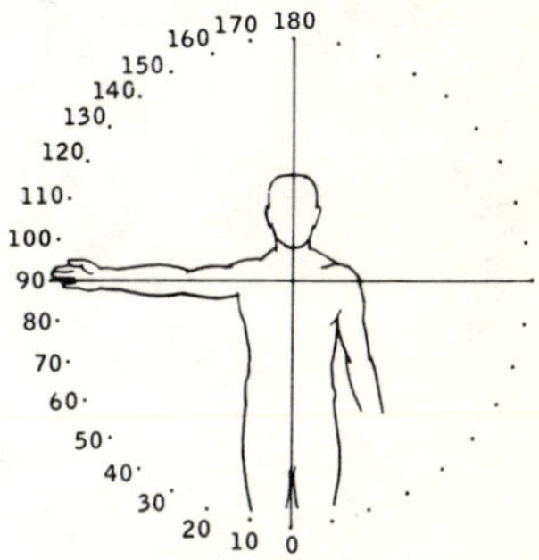

Figure 30. Recording R.O.M. chart of shoulder and scapula with rotary scapula movements.

that are most commonly injured. I hope that these charts will be of value to the reader. By comparing the normal ranges with the ones of the injured athlete, you will hopefully be able to establish an evaluation of injury and, furthermore, provide better care.

7. Testing Muscle Strength

Strength of a muscle or a group of muscles is determined by manual muscle testing. Manual muscle testing is usually performed by the physical therapist, who has considerable knowledge of the origin and insertion of each muscle as well as the action of each muscle. Manual muscle testing permits one to evaluate the strength of a movement. The evaluation of testing muscle strength requires the ability to isolate, eliminate, and stabilize the joint in such a way that the desirable movement is performed. For example, the gastrocnemius attach the condyles of the femur; it is possible to eliminate the role of that muscle considerably by testing plantar flexion with the knee flexed. In this way, the strength of the soleus can be tested, although the gastrocnemius still makes some contribution. The strength of each movement is graded from 0 to 5, from absent to normal. Below there is a chart illustrating this point.

Table I

Grade	Muscular contraction	Definition
0	absent	no muscular contraction
1	trace	minimal contraction; no joint motion
2	poor	R.O.M. complete when gravity eliminated
3	fair	R.O.M. complete against gravity
4	good	R.O.M. complete against gravity but not strong enough to overcome resistance appropriate for age, sex, and occupation.
5	normal	R.O.M. complete against gravity and strong enough to overcome resistance appropriate for age, sex, and occupation.

I have briefly discussed the topic of muscle strength so that the reader will be able to follow the terminology used by physicians, physical therapists, and other professionals during the evaluation of an injury.

Table II

LOWER EXTREMITIES

DATE

DATE

			L	R	L	R
Hip						
1. Flexion (bent knee)	0	115				
2. Flexion (straight leg)	0	80				
3. Extension	0	15				
4. Abduction	0	45				
5. Adduction	45	0				
6. Internal rotation	0	45				
7. External rotation	0	45				
Knee						
1. Flexion	0	125				
2. Extension	125	0				
Foot						
1. Dorsi flexion	0	20				
2. Plantar flexion	0	45				

UPPER EXTREMITIES

DATE

DATE

Shoulder		
1. Flexion	0	90
2. Extension	0	50
3. Abduction	0	90
4. Adduction	90	0
5. External rotation	0	90
6. Internal rotation	0	90
Elbow		
1. Flexion	0	145
2. Extension	145	0
3. Supination	0	90
4. Pronation	0	90

Table II (continued)

Range of motion of the lower and upper extremities

Wrist				L	R	L	R
1. Flexion		0	90				
2. Extension		0	70				
Fingers							
1. M. P. flexion	1 & 2						
0 90	3 & 4						
2. M. P. extension	1 & 2						
0 25	3 & 4						
3. Prox. I.P. flexion	1 & 2						
0 120	3 & 4						
4. Prox. I.P. extension	1 & 2						
120 0	3 & 4						
5. Dist. I.P. flexion	1 & 2						
0 75	3 & 4						
6. Dist. I.P. extension	1 & 2						
75 0	3 & 4						
Thumb							
1. M.P. flexion		0	60				
2. Extension		60	0				
3. I.P. flexion		0	90				
4. Extension		90	0				

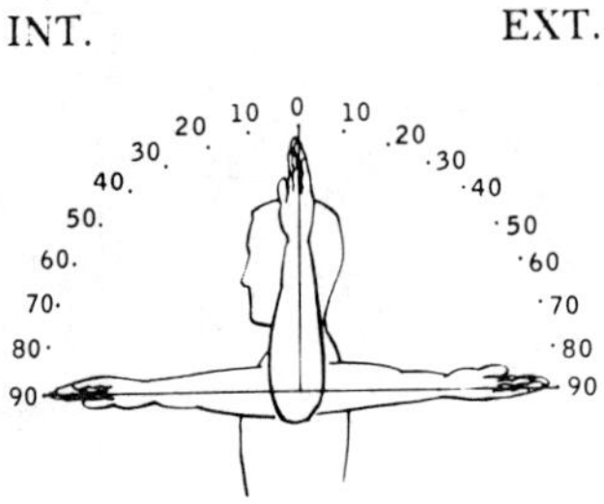

SHOULDER ROTATION

Elbow flexed		90
Ext. Rot.	0 –	90
Int. Rot.	0 –	90

LIMITATIONS

	L		R	
	Int.	Ext.	Int.	Ext.
1				
2				
3				
4				

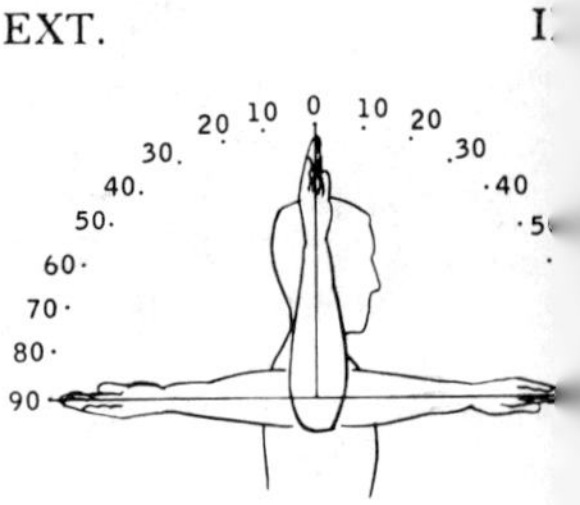

Figure 31. Chart for recording the range of motion of the shoulder.

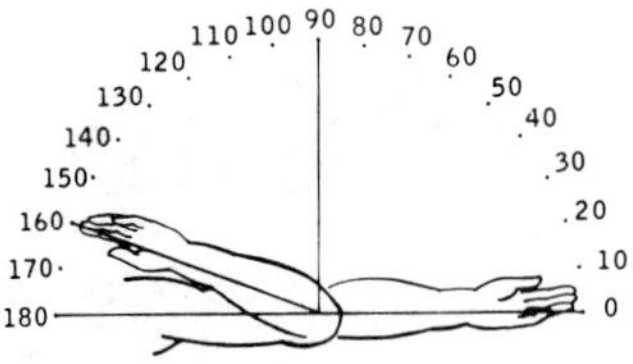

ELBOW

Flexion	0 –	145 –	160
Extension	160 –	145 –	0

LIMITATIONS

	L		R	
	Flex.	Ext.	Flex.	Ext.
1				
2				
3				
4				

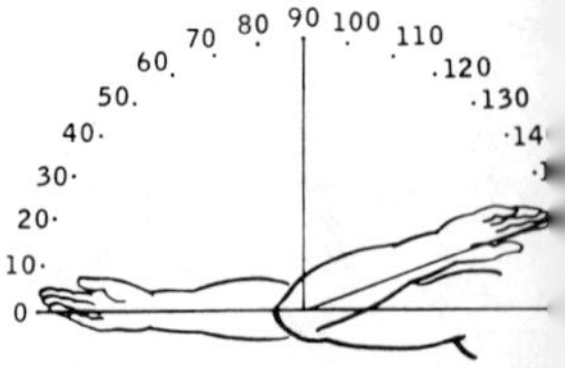

Figure 32. Chart for recording the range of motion of the elbow.

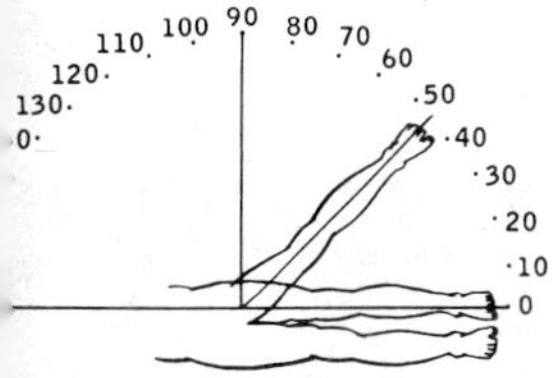

HIP

Abduction		0 – 45	
Adduction		0 – 45	

LIMITATIONS

L		R	
Abd.	Add.	Abd.	Add.
1			
2			
3			
4			

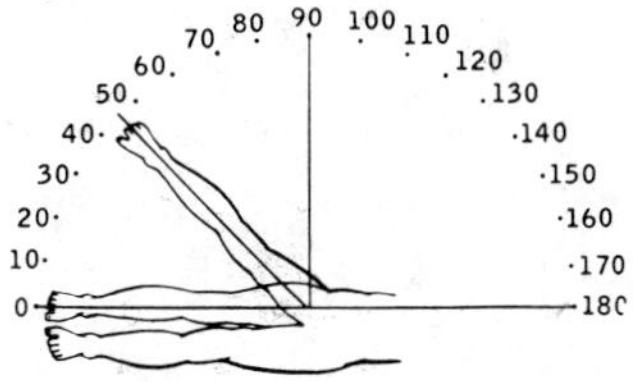

EXT.

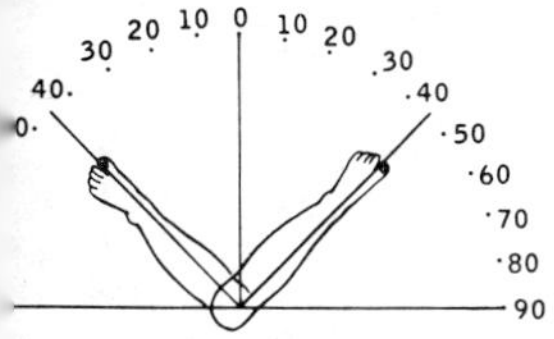

HIP (BENT KNEE PRONE)

Ext. Rot.		0 – 45	
Int. Rot.		0 – 45	

LIMITATIONS

L		R	
Int.	Ext.	Int.	Ext.
1			
2			
3			
4			

EXT. INT.

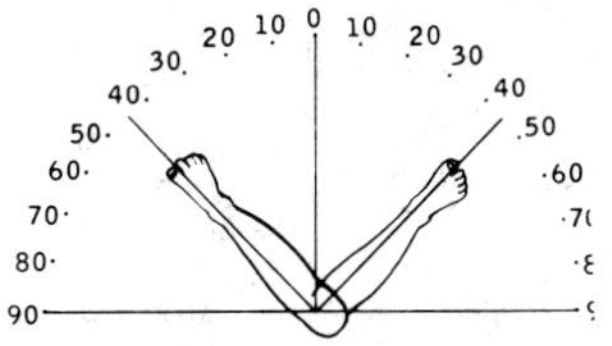

KNEE

Flex. (prone)	0 – 120 – 130		
Extension	130 – 120 – 0		

LIMITATIONS

L		R	
Fl.	Ext.	Fl.	Ext.
1			
2			
3			
4			

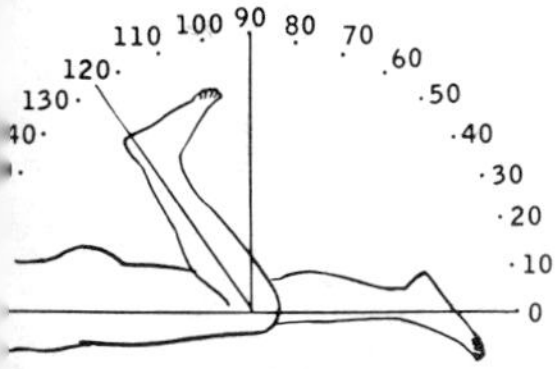

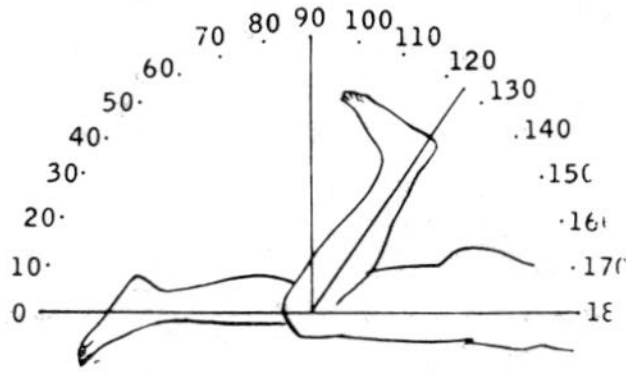

NTAR DORSAL

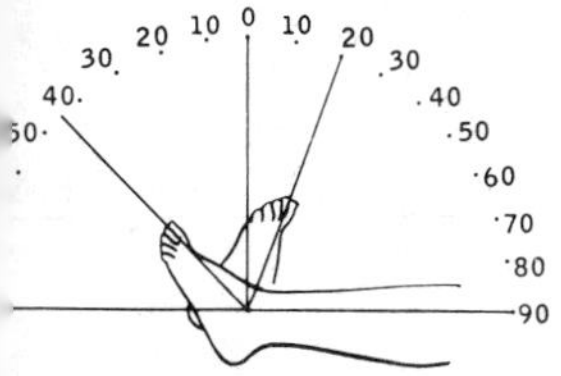

ANKLE

Flexion		0 – 20	
Extension		0 – 45	

LIMITATIONS

L		R	
Fl.	Ext.	Fl.	Ext.
1			
2			
3			
4			

DORSAL PLANTAR

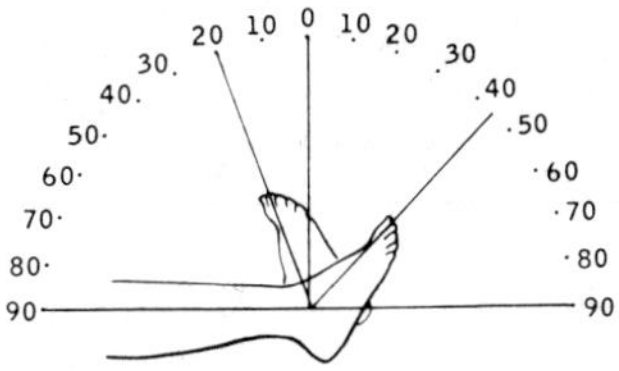

Figure 33. Chart for recording the range of motion of the hip, knee, and ankle.

HIP

Fl. (str. knee)	0 – 90
Fl. (bent knee)	0 – 115 – 125
Extension	0 – 10 – 15
Ext. & lumbar spine	0 – 15 – 45

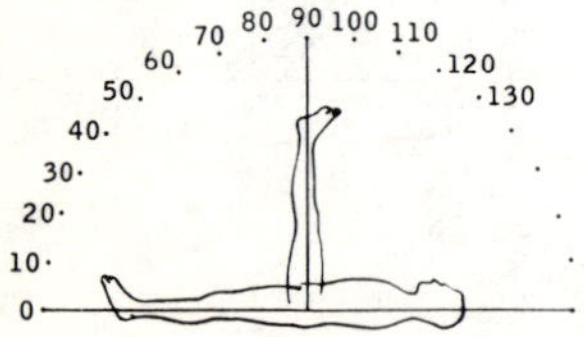

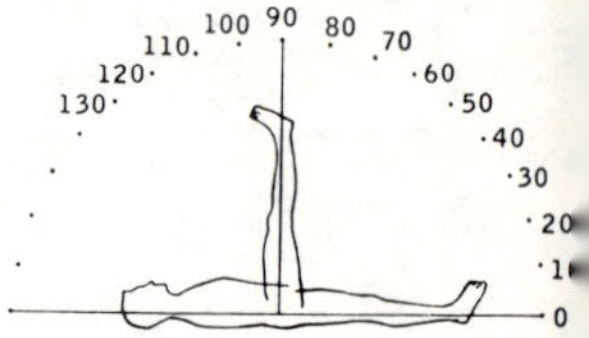

LIMITATIONS
FLEXION (Straight Knee)

	L		R	
	Fl.	Ext.	Fl.	Ext.
1				
2				
3				
4				

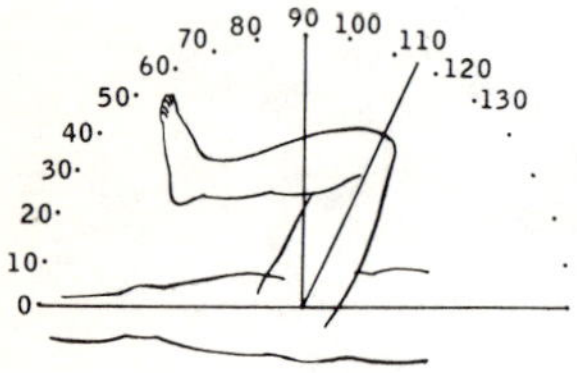

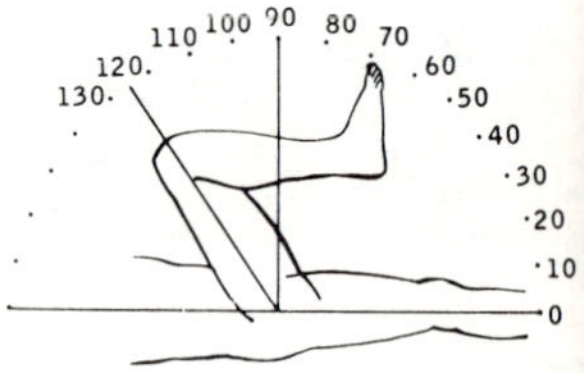

FLEXION (BENT KNEE)

	L		R	
	Fl.	Ext.	Fl.	Ext.
1				
2				
3				
4				

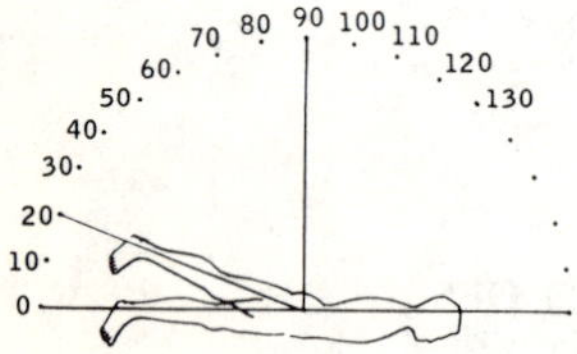

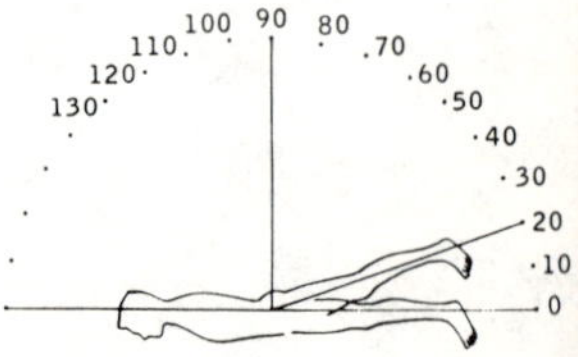

EXTENSION

	L		R	
	Ext.	E. & L.	Ext.	E. & L.
1				
2				
3				
4				

Figure 34. Chart for recording the range of motion of the hip, knee, and ankle.

PART II
BODILY INJURIES IN ORDER OF OCCURRENCE

8. Knee Injuries and Care

General Discussion (Figures 35-39)

The knee joint is a hinge joint, forming the articulation between the lower end of the femur or thigh bone and the upper end of the tibia. The fibula and the patella also complete the bone structure of the joint. A hinge joint allows two basic movements, flexion and extension about a horizontal axis; however, in view of the shapes of the articular surfaces, these movements are combined with gliding and rolling as well as rotary movements about a vertical axis. The combined movements of this highly sophisticated joint makes it highly susceptible to injury and, consequently, pain. Pain following injury to the knee is manifested through an amazingly complicated plexus of nerves, that supply all structures in and around the joint. In view of this intricate neuromuscular mechanism and its relationship with all tissues that make the knee joint work, the pain that is felt leads to "favoring the part," and, as an end result, the quadriceps that activate the knee begin to atrophy (weaken).

General Signs and Symptoms After Knee Injury

1. Pain
2. Swelling
3. "Water on the knee"
4. Locking
5. "Knee gives away"
6. "Pinching" felt inside the knee
7. Limitation of R.O.M. (range of motion or movement)
8. Tenderness
9. Muscle weakness
10. Discoloration

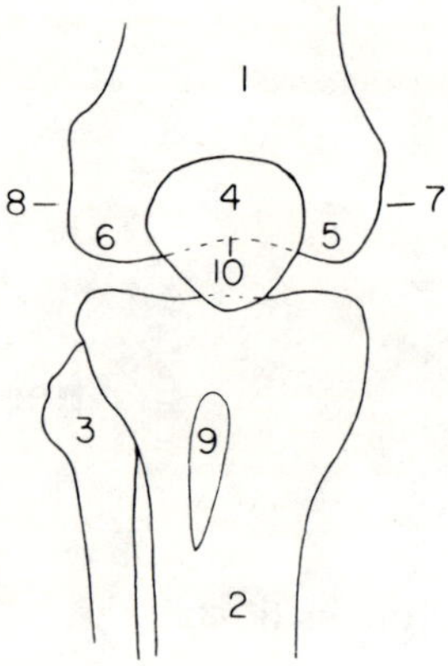

Figure 35. Anatomical landmarks of the knee joint. 1. Femur; 2. Tibia; 3. Fibula; 4. Patella; 5. Medial Condyle; 6. Lateral Condyle; 7. Medial Epicondyle; 8. Lateral Epicondyle; 9. Tibial Tubercle; 10. Intercondylar Notch.

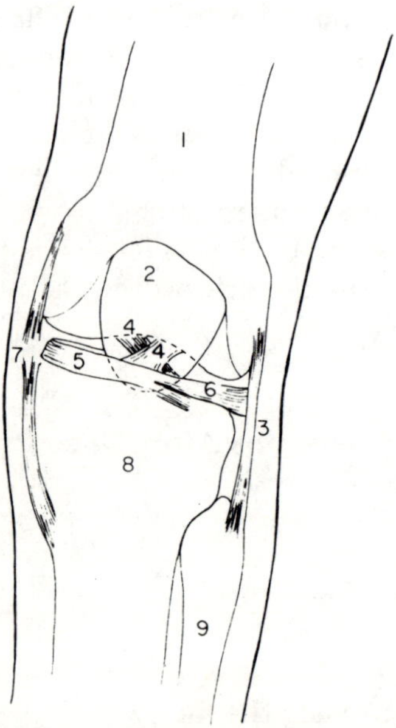

Figure 36. Anatomical attachments. 1. Femur; 2. Patella; 3. Lateral collateral ligament; 4. Cruciate ligaments; 5. Medial Meniscus; 6. Lateral Meniscus; 7. Ruptured Medial Col ligament; 8. Tibia, 9. Fibula; 10. Anterior Cruciate ligament; 11. Torn medial Meniscus; 12. Posterior Cruciate ligament

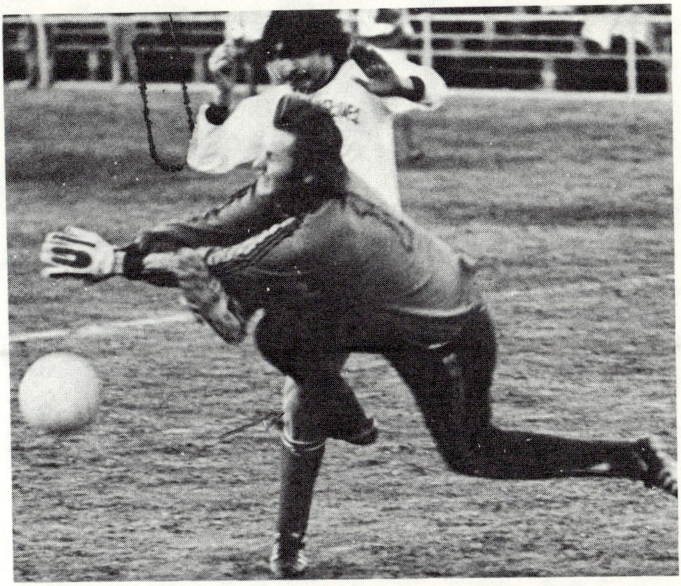

Figure 36a. Possible Site of Medial Knee-joint injury. Forces applied indicated by arrow result in injury to (1) medial collateral) (2) medial meniscus; (3) cruciate ligaments.

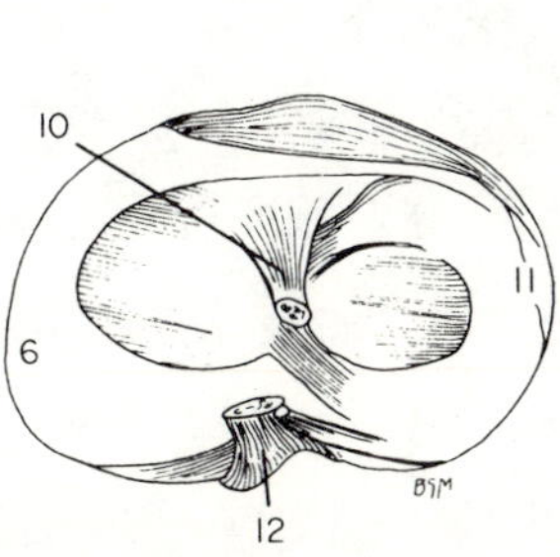

Figure 37. Tibial, plateau (from above).

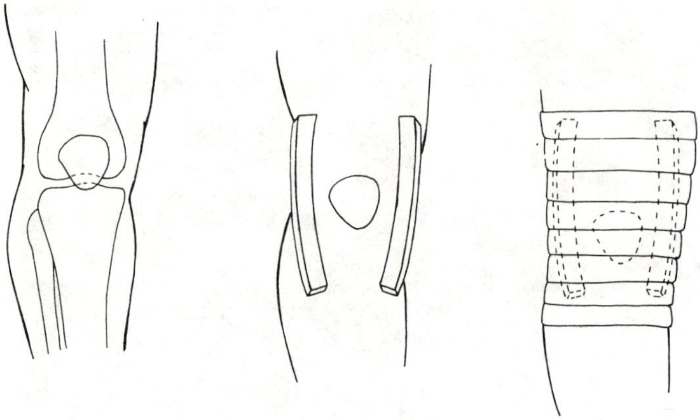

Figure 38a, b. Anterior anatomical structures of the knee; a) two strips of firm felt material pointed by arrows; b) complete strapping of the knee joint for medio-lateral support.

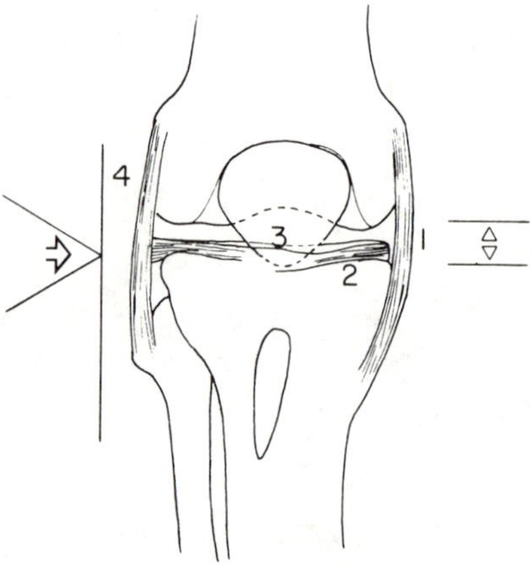

Figure 38c. Arrow points out the force that results in injury to medial collateral ligament. Other structures are: 2) medial meniscus; 3) cruciate ligament; 4) lateral collateral ligament.

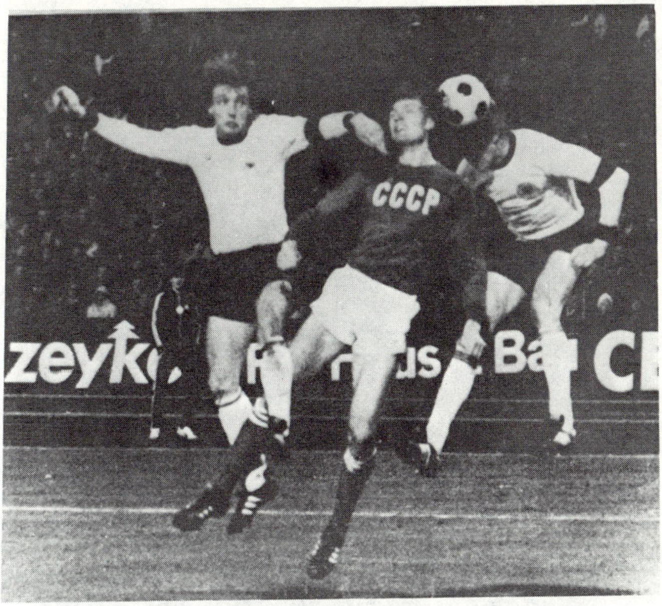

Figure 38d. Possible Site of Injury of the Lateral Cartilage of the Right Knee. Site shown by arrows.

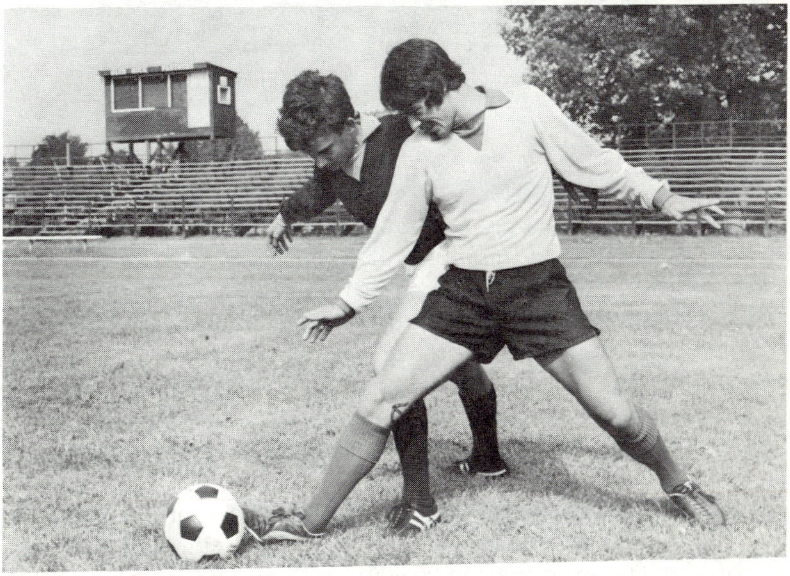

Figure 38e. Possible Site of Medial Collateral Ligament Knee Injury.

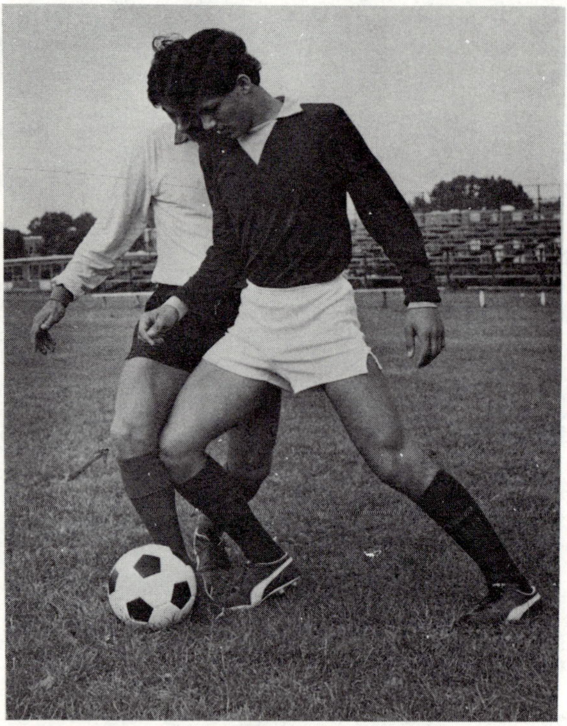

Figure 38f. Possible Site of Lateral Collateral Ligament Injury.

11. Crepitus (cracking at joint during movement)
12. Insecurity and limping
13. Clicking or grating sound heard or felt
14. Change of shape, especially the circumference of the knee

Upon examination of the knee joint, the soccer player must give you a complete detailed history of the accident, revealing the incidents that resulted in his condition. Each detail must be noted and utilized into the athlete's immediate and postcare. After the long, detailed description of the knee injury, it will be wise to ask information regarding previous injuries to the knee. Quite often there may have been injuries that were considered insignificant but should nevertheless not be ignored in the examination as well as future rehabilitative care. In examining knee injuries, the following priorities must apply:

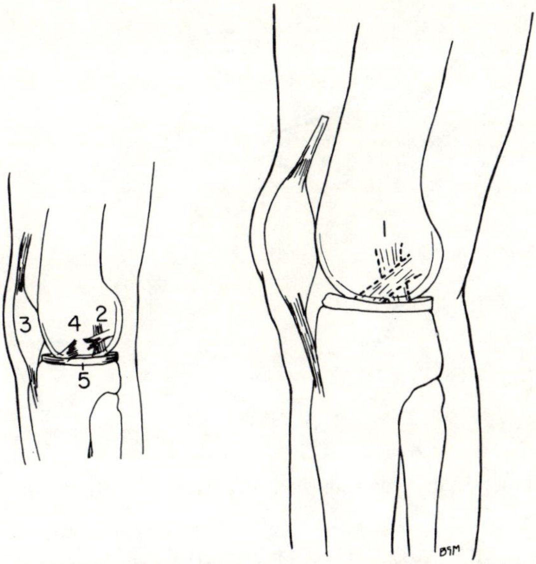

Figure 39. Side view of normal knee joint. 1. Normal Cruciate Ligaments; 2. Posterior Cruciate; 3. Patella; 4. Ruptured Anterior Cruciate; 5. Lateral Meniscus.

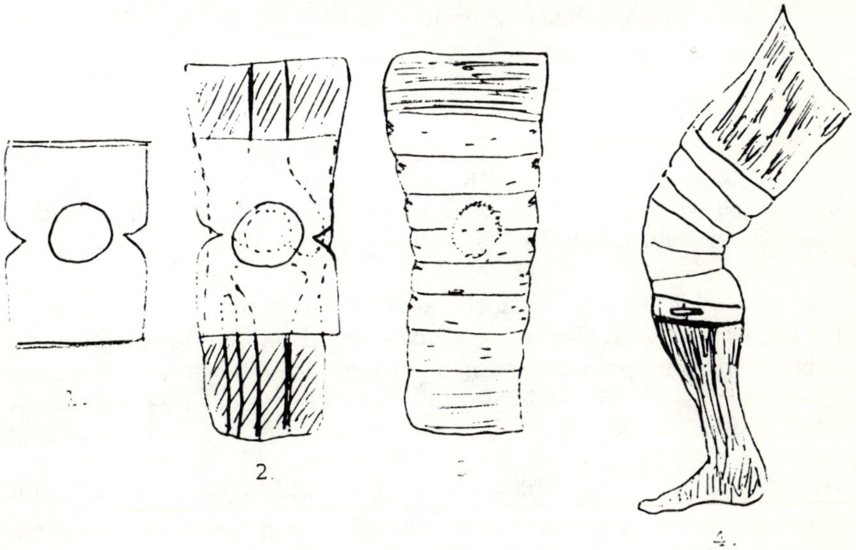

Figure 39a. Medial collateral strapping with sponge rubber.

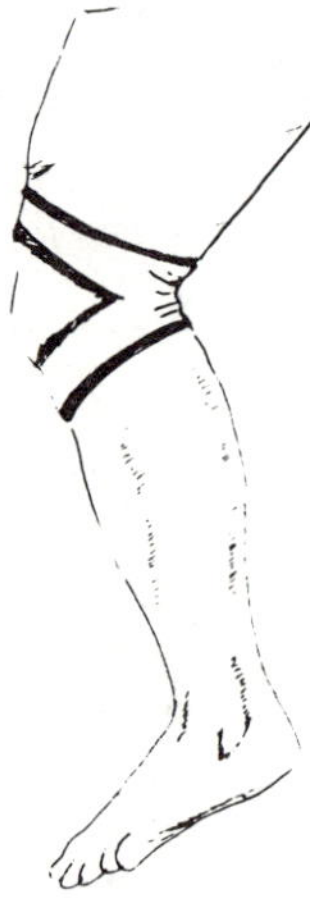

Figure 39b. Knee strapping for hyperextension knee injury.

1. Relieve pain, apply cold packs to all knee injuries.
2. Keep athlete prone or on his stomach.
3. Be aware of the possibility of athlete going into shock.
4. Keep athlete warm.
5. Examine him very slowly; no sudden movements.
6. Ask questions for player's reactions to his injury.
7. Ask for ambulance when in dilemma.

Diagnostic Tests

In the process of examination, the following functional tests should be applied while the athlete is flat on his back. These tests should be applied very cautiously.

Flexion and Extension. With the athlete flat on his back, grasp lower leg firmly and bend the knee as far as it will go. Should you meet any oppositions (i.e., pain, stiffness, tightness), investigate why the opposition is present. Proceed the same for full extension as illustrated. (Figure 40a)

Lateral Instability Test. With the leg in full extension, grasp the ankle with one hand and place the other hand around the lower part of the posterior thigh. By holding the thigh firm, gently pull the lower leg toward you; this will open the joint. Should motion occur, check the

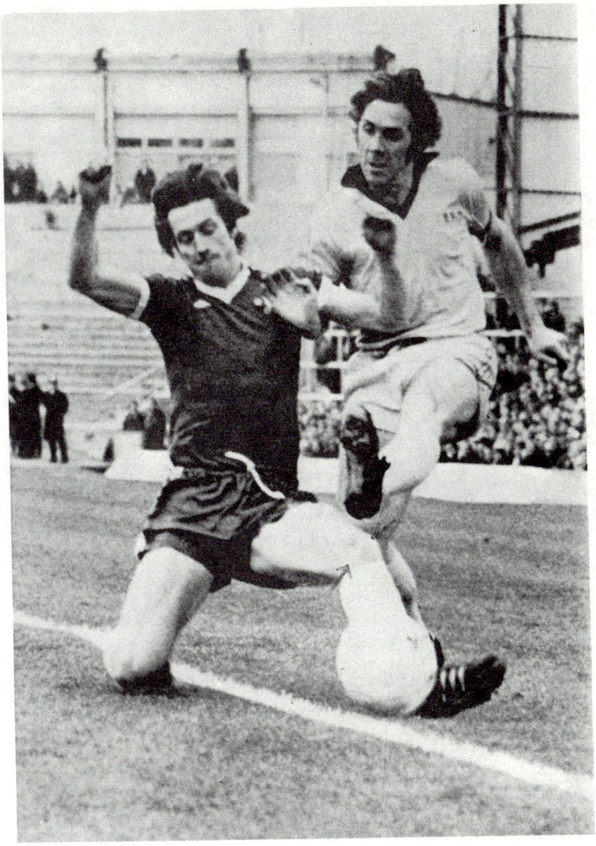

Figure 39c. Possible Sites of Lateral, Collateral and Cruciate Ligaments (Posterior).

other knee joint in the same manner. This is to test the stability of the medial collateral ligament; reverse the process for the lateral collateral ligament. Testing the amount of instability in full extension, there should be no movement. If movement exists, there must be some ligamentous tear, and the soccer player must be referred to the orthopedic surgeon. (Figures 40c, d)

Cruciate Ligaments. These can be tested by flexing the knee and placing the ankle under your arm, locking it in place with your elbow. Both hands then are placed around the upper part of the lower leg, with the thumbs upward on the tibial tubercle. Then press down for testing the posterior cruciate and pull forward for testing the anterior

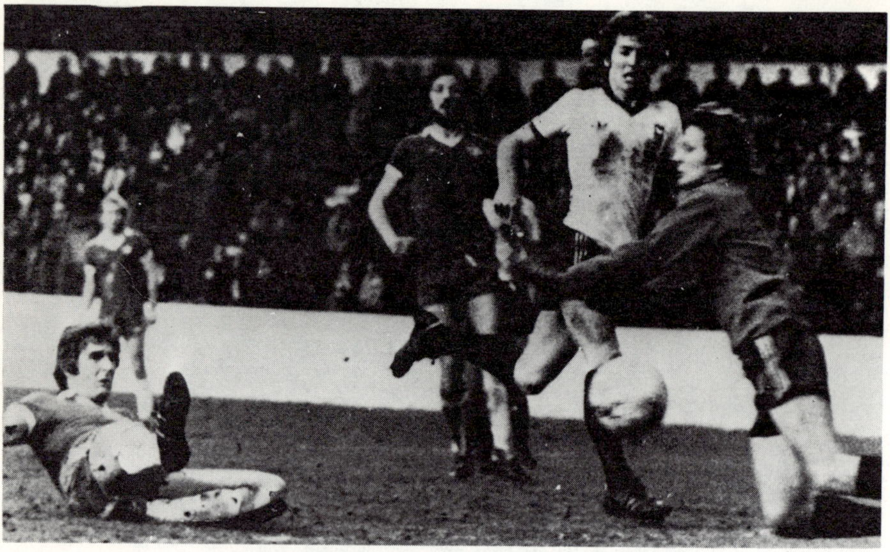

Figure 39d. Possible site of Anterior Cruciate Ligament Injury.

cruciate. The riding forward or backward of the knee joint will indicate slack of cruciate ligaments. (Figure 40)

When the treatment has been decided, it should be applied as soon after the injury as possible, not the next day, but even on the soccer field at the time of the injury. For example, if the player has to apply to his knee an ice pack, compression bandage, and elevation, do so immediately by making these adaptations on the soccer field or by driving the player to his home if above adaptations are not possible. Do not wait until the match is over and then proceed with treatment. Treatments to be used are decided on as soon as possible and then carried out to their entirety (completion).

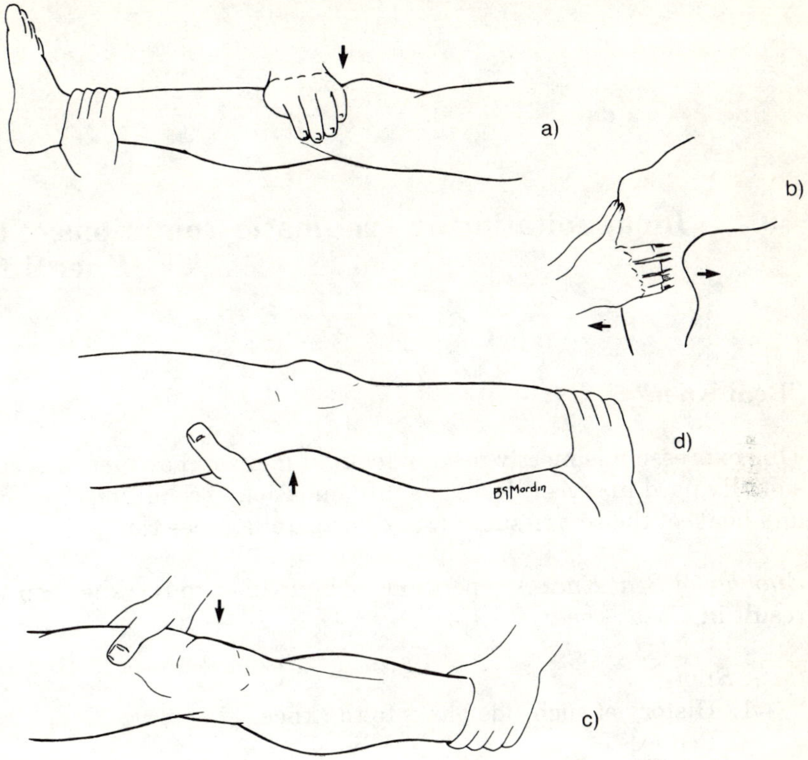

Figure 40. a) test for full extension; b) test for the anterior and posterior cruciates; c) test for lateral collateral; d) test for medial collateral.

9. Incapacitating or Traumatic Conditions of the Knee Joint

"Beat Knee"

This expression is mostly used in football injuries; however, it is ocassionally used in soccer. It means inflammation (a condition of redness and heat) of the soft tissues around the patella (knee cap).

Etiology of Beat Knee A repetitious oblique blow to the knee cap will result in a beat knee.

Basic Signs:

1. History of such side blows to the knee
2. Redness
3. Minor swelling
4. Dull ache
5. Tenderness to touch

Treatment

1. Application of cold packs around the knee joint for 30-minute intervals, throughout 24-hour period.
2. Protective knee strapping 3–6 inches above and below the knee.
3. Continue this protection even when the player is capable of attending practice.
4. Application of whirlpool after 24 hours, at 102–104° F.
5. Progressive resistive exercises to the quadriceps after the third or fourth day, depending on the severity of the injury. The lesser the degree of injury, the sooner the intensity of exercise should begin. In this case, by the third day, progressive exercise will not harm the knee. Usually by the third or fourth day, the athlete can return to practice.

"Buckle Knee"

It is a condition by which the knee can not maintain the "anatomic stability" and "gives away" under exhaustion. It happens usually near the end of the game to athletes who haven't attended practice sessions during the week. During exhaustion, the quadriceps relax and the knee collapses. All muscles and other soft tissues "let go" simultaneously.

Etiology

1. Fatigue
2. Mental exhaustion or emotional stress
3. Dietary deficiency
4. Old knee injuries without proper care of the quadriceps
5. Cartilage damage
6. Weight imbalance from foot problems resulting from improper shoes

Treatment

1. Moist heat application.
2. Whirlpool.
3. Progressive resistive exercises to quadriceps and often Hamstrings.
4. Check shoes and arch support; sometimes a lift on the heel or on the ball of foot might prevent this condition.
5. Check player for any emotional problem.

Cartilage Injuries

Cartilage injuries often are mistaken when, in fact, collateral ligaments are torn. Quite often, however, a combination of both may occur. When this happens, the time of disability overextends to perhaps several months, and quite often the player may not return to the soccer field unless the proper surgical procedure is followed by rehabilitation techniques. Under cartilage injuries, we have two types: medial cartilage (meniscus) and lateral cartilage (meniscus). The former one (medial) is the most common one, and it will be discussed first.

Medial Cartilage (meniscus) Injuries. This type of injury is most frequent possibly because the chances of getting a blow from the outside of the knee are much greater than getting the same from the inside. This outside forceful blow causes internal derangement to the knee joint by forcefully rotating inwardly the femur on the tibia and abducting (throwing outwardly) the lower leg. The same force, resulting from a blow coming from inside to the knee joint while the knee is somewhat flexed, causes a lateral cartilage injury. The same type of injury might result when the athlete lands on uneven ground, deranging the knee joint internally cr externally (Figures 35–39, Chapter 8).

It must be emphasized that knee injuries are caused most of the time, in fact, all the time, when the knee is partly flexed and twisted outwardly or inwardly, depending on the situation. When this occurs, the cartilage splits or tears. In view of the poor circulation of this area, the healing is very slow even on healthy athletes. When orthopedic surgery is ruled out, and/or when the cartilage is removed surgically, physical therapy plays a very important role in rehabilitating the knee joint, and its surrounding tissues.

Basic Signs and Symptoms

1. Functional tests to be carried out in the field if possible.
2. Limitation of extension of the knee joint.
3. McMurray's sign is a valuable asset to know in establishing a diagnosis—place hand over the joint; a click will be felt when the tibia moves; the click may be heard as well.
4. Reduce the dislocation (should be done under the direction of a physician or the physician himself). In recurring instances, the athlete manipulates the reduction himself.

Treatment (Immediately after injury)

1. Application of cold packs.
2. Posterior splint, keeping knee in full extension or as much as it allows at this point without much discomfort.
3. Compression bandage extending 10–15 inches above and below the knee joint.
4. Medcollator (muscle stimulation) within the limits of comfort.
5. Knee elevation while athlete is lying on his back (supine).

6. Active movement of the ankle joint as well as straight leg raising should be emphasized to prevent any atrophy that might occur from disuse above and below the knee joint.

Treatment after 48 hours

1. Hydrocollator hot packs.
2. Medcollator.
3. Active assistive movement of the knee joint in flexion and extension.
4. Quadriceps—setting exercises (tighten the knee cap, no joint movement).
5. Strapping of the knee joint should be applied for walking, if so permitted by the orthopedic surgeon, using flexible straps extending 10 inches above and below the knee joint. Special wrapping material should be applied over the same length before strapping to avoid hair pulling (Figures 26 and 39b).
6. Teach athlete crutch walking should weight bearing not be permitted by orthopedic surgeon.
7. When weight bearing is allowed and resistive movements permitted, teach athlete a progressive resistive exercise program (discussed in another chapter in greater detail) to build up his muscles surrounding the knee joint with emphasis on his quadriceps.
8. The application of isokinetics to build up the quadriceps. (Isokinetics will be discussed in greater detail in another chapter.)

Long Range Treatment. When there is no evidence of swelling, pain, and the range of movement of the knee joint is complete, the player should attend practice sessions in the following manner:

1. Stretching—attempt slowly to touch your toes by keeping the knees straight. Do not bounce up and down to accomplish it. One downward slow movement to be maintained for 20 seconds should be enough.
2. Repeat above 5 times.
3. Keep feet together while body erect in a standing position and attempt to lift knee to chest alternately.
4. Begin walking slowly the length of the field, progressing to maximum walking speed until completion of field's circumference.
5. Begin jogging, completing half the field's circumference; progress to comfortable acceleration and to maximum acceleration for the last 50 feet.

6. Third time around, comfortable accelerating speed with maximum acceleration every 20 yards until field's circumference is completed.

7. Proceed to a comfortable speed in a winding path, progressing to maximum speed at intervals of 10 yards alternately, between comfortable and maximum speeds, respectively.

Note: The player should have a protective flexible strapping while above procedure is applied.

8. Upon completion of above procedure, the player should remove the strapping and proceed with hot and cold compresses to the knee joint, for 20 minutes to an hour.

9. Upon completion, the elastic strapping should be reapplied if an active working day is anticipated.

10. At night, the strapping should be removed unless the athlete feels more comfortable with it.

Lateral Cartilage Meniscus. This is subject to the same type of injury as the medial meniscus; however, it is less frequent, and the incidence is about 1 in 10. Pain and other signs and symptoms will be the same except on the lateral side (outside) of the knee joint. This injury, although it occurs less frequently than the medial injury, is, nevertheless, just as disabling. The method of immediate and long-range treatment is exactly the same as for the medial cartilage.

Medial Collateral Ligament (Fig. 38c, Chapter 8)

Injury to this ligament is very common in soccer. This type of injury is often mistaken with injury to the medial meniscus. If this injury is too severe, however, the medial meniscus may be involved as well. The medial collateral ligament is attached at the femoral epicondyle and the medial condyle of the tibia, and partly to the medial meniscus. It is a short, fat, and broad ligament whose main function is to protect the knee joint's medial aspect as well as assisting the function of medial meniscus. See Figure 38e, Chapter 8. The arrow points out the force that results in injury to: (1) medial collateral ligament, (2) medial meniscus, (3) cruciate ligaments, (4) lateral collateral ligament.

Etiology: The most common cause is a hit on the lateral aspect of the knee with the foot planted on the ground. This motion causes the medial aspect to enlarge, thus stretching the medial collateral ligament.

Basic Signs and Symptoms

Mild Injury to Medial Collateral

1. Insecurity of the knee joint
2. Minor tear of the ligament
3. Tenderness on the medial aspect when walking and/or running
4. When abducting the tibia
5. Mild pain when repeated motion

Moderate Injury to Medial Collateral

1. Considerable and obvious insecurity of the knee
2. Partial tear of the ligament
3. Tenderness even when standing
4. Localized swelling with diffusion
5. A lot of pain when repeated motion

Severe Injury to Medial Collateral

1. Total insecurity of the knee joint.
2. Severe abduction of the lower leg plus rotation, forcing the ligament to go beyond its normal range.
3. In such severe injuries, there will be damage to one or more ligaments and the medial meniscus.
4. Increased localized swelling.
5. Normal contours of the knee as compared with the other may appear to be obliterated by the swelling.
6. There may be a locking of joint indicating cartilage involvement.
7. Extension will be markedly impaired.

Treatment of Medial Collateral Injury

Mild

1. Application of ice packs.
2. Compression ace bandage extending several inches above and below the joint. (Apply ace bandage from below and move upwards.)
3. Elevation—lying on back, elevate knee above shoulder level.
4. After 24 hours, apply moist heat and/or whirlpool followed by active movements in flexion and extension.
5. The third day, apply resistance to the quadriceps. (See progressive resistive exercises in an earlier chapter.)

6. Strapping or bandaging will depend on the player.

Moderate (after the physician has ruled out fracture)

1. Compression with an elastic adhesive.
2. Ice-pack application.
3. Elevation.
4. Reinforcement of the elastic adhesive with 12-inch sponge rubber with a hole at the center to encompass the patella. See Fig. 39a showing *compression wrap of knee*: (1) sponge rubber cut to form of knee; (2) application of rubber to knee; (3) compression wrap of elastic bandage applied very snugly over the rubber; (4) apply reinforcement bandage with the knee semiflexed.

Severe

Note: all moderate and severe injuries should be x-rayed routinely.

1. Immediate care should be exactly the same as in moderate, that is, compression, ice pack, elevation, and bed rest.
2. A splint should be applied posteriorly, conforming to the contours of the knee, maintaining the knee in approximately 30 degrees of flexion.

Note: Elastic ace bandages, elastic adhesive tapes, felt strips, and other materials have been discussed in an earlier chapter.

3. The use of crutches to eliminate weight bearing the first two to three days will be very helpful and will accelerate restoration of the injury.
4. After 48 hours, apply moist heat under and over the knee joint using hydrocollator hot packs.
5. Medcollator at this time will be very helpful in preventing muscle atrophy.
6. Quadriceps setting exercises
7. Progressive resistive exercises starting without any weight and progressing to maximum load, is very essential for the rehabilitation of the knee.
8. Maximum results will be obtained when the involved knee will be compatible with the noninvolved knee.
9. Begin jogging for 10 yards, progressing to walking 20 yards, and then accelerate progressively in a straight line.
10. When the player is capable of alternately jogging and sprinting in a straight line and in a winding or zig-zag path, then he is ready to attend practice.

Note: A severe injury, such as the above, will take at least a few months to be restored, depending on the repair process of the player's ligament plus the condition of his quadriceps.

Lateral Collateral Ligament

The lateral collateral ligament is situated at the lateral epicondyle of the femur and bridges over the lateral aspect of the joint to the head of the fibula. (Figure 38c)

This ligament is not attached to the lateral cartilage; therefore, severe injuries of this ligament do not involve the lateral meniscus or cartilage. Consequently, this injury is not as disabling as the medial collateral. Injury to this ligament is very uncommon since a direct blow to the medial side forcing the lateral side to split very rarely is seen. In the mild and moderate type of injuries to this ligament the immediate treatment will be the same as for the medial collateral:

1. compression
2. ice
3. elevation

Note: Neither muscle atrophy nor tenderness and swelling are noted in lateral collateral, as it is in medial collateral.

In severe injury, posterior splint is indicated initially—when surgery is ruled out by the orthopedic surgeon—as well as crutch walking to eliminate weight bearing and accelerate restoration. The rehabilitation of the quadriceps is very important because a strong quadriceps group will reduce the chances of repetitious injury to this ligament. The rehabilitation time and the return of the player to the field is much shorter—usually within two months—provided physical therapy is carried out regularly with progressive resistive exercises to the quadriceps and the use of other modalities.

Hyperextension Knee Injuries

This type of injury occurs when the knee joint extends beyond its normal range of extension, consequently, stretching the muscles that ordinarily flex the knee. In moderate to severe injuries, it is possible to see partial ligamentous tear as well.

Etiology. This type of injury occurs most commonly under three different conditions of action as follows:

1. When the player lands to the ground on his heels, forcing both knees to go backwards.

2. When a player is kicked or pushed on one or both knees while his feet are planted on the ground.

3. When a player attempts to hit a ground ball very hard and he misses.

Basic Signs and Symptoms

1. Dull pain on the back of his knee.

2. Instability of the knee joint upon bearing weight, especially when standing on the injured knee.

3. Tenderness will be present at the lower attachments of the hamstrings and the upper attachment of the calf muscles.

4. Pain and tenderness will be felt more when the knee is in extension.

Treatment of Hyperextension injuries

1. Immediate treatment with the application of ice packs, compression, and elevation.

2. Adhesive elastic strapping application with the knee positioned at 10–15 degrees of flexion (Figure 39b).

3. After 24–36 hours, apply moist heat and/or whirlpool to 106° F.

4. Electrical stimulation for 5 to 8 minutes is helpful before progressive resistive exercise begins.

5. Active movements emphasizing complete R.O.M. (range of motion): in this case, complete knee extension is indicated.

6. Apply a ¾-inch lift under the heel. This lift will force the knee into some flexion, thus reducing discomfort from pain during walking.

7. Using the quadriceps table (or N/K table) begin P.R.E. (progressive resistive exercises), starting with quads, for the purpose of relaxing the hamstrings, and then proceed P.R.E. with the hamstrings. The player should alternate while applying P.R.E. techniques to strengthen both groups, the quadriceps and the hamstrings. In the case of hyperextension, the emphasis should be placed in strengthening the hamstrings.

Note: The above treatment should be applied every day of the week. Once the R.O.M. has been complete, and the pain and tenderness have subsided during exercise, the player should attempt practice sessions on the soccer field. This injury in a well-trained athlete does not take more than 3–4 days before complete recovery.

Cruciate Ligaments Injury

The cruciate ligaments are very important ligaments of the knee joint. They are very short and very strong ligaments whose function is not only to stabilize the knee in the anterior and posterior motion of the tibia, as many authors point out, but also to limit outward rotation of the femur (thigh bone) upon the tibia. Their anatomical attachments, in crossing the tibia and femur, will point out clearly their functions (Figure 36a). The anterior cruciate ligament is usually injured when the knee is forced to go into hyperextension. The anterior cruciate will also tear when there is a severe injury to the medial collateral ligament. Any severe injury, therefore, of the anterior cruciate must be accompanied, in most cases, by an injury of the medial collateral and/or the medial meniscus (cartilage). The posterior cruciate ligament is usually injured when the knee is flexed beyond its normal limits or hyperflexed. A violent wrenching of the knee, however, will not only damage the posterior cruciate, but, as a rule, it will damage the anterior cruciate as well.

Signs and Symptoms of Cruciate Injury

1. Pain and loss of function.
2. Instability: "the knee feels like its giving under."
3. Swelling.
4. Tenderness during functional test examinations.
5. Depending which cruciate, tenderness will also be present on the medial or lateral collateral attachments.

Note: Functional tests for collateral ligaments, medial and lateral menisci, and cruciate ligaments have been described earlier in this chapter.

Treatment of Cruciate ligaments

1. As a routine, the player must be taken for x-rays, which, in fact, will show nothing except to rule out any possibility of fracture.
2. Immediate care with the application of ice packs, compression bandage, and elevation even before the player sees a physician.

3. In a severe injury resulting in torn cruciate ligaments, splinting of the knee joint from the lower leg to the upper thigh is advocated. The splinting is preferable to casting because it can be removed, adjusted, and reapplied while, at the same time, mild active assistive R.O.M. can be very beneficial. In addition, the active movement of the knee will eliminate any possible atrophy that might have resulted if cast was applied.

4. After the splint is applied, the player will be on crutches, and he must be taught to walk without bearing weight on his injured leg.

5. When the splint is removed, and partial weight bearing is allowed, a progressive resistive exercise program should begin.

Note: Players who have been treated conservatively with full cast, take much longer to come to the stage where R.O.M. has been completed and extensive P.R.E. begins.

6. Moist heat (hydrocollator hot packs) applied to both surfaces should precede the P.R.E.

7. After severe injury, it will take the player approximately 8–10 weeks before he returns to the soccer field. The exercise routine to follow once on the soccer field should be the same as the one described in postmeniscus injury earlier in this chapter.

Special Notation: The soccer player must be aware of the fact that the thigh muscles are the ones that guard the knee. Any weakness resulting from disuse will directly affect the knee joint. The most important muscles the soccer player has are the quadriceps—the rectus femuris, the vastus medialis, the vastus lateralis, and vastus intermedius. These muscles are the "watchdog of the knee and the guardian of the ligaments." It is, therefore, of the utmost importance that physical therapy in the form of progressive resistive exercise begins as soon as the immediate care has been given and as soon as active movement is possible. The recognition of the restoration of this group of muscles should be the immediate concern of the coach and trainer. Atrophy of the quadriceps indicates inability to participate in soccer.

Osgood-Schlatter's Disease

I am mentioning this disease because many high-school athletes and some from college were very much concerned when pain developed just below the patella. The pain increased when the knee was forced in flexion and/or when resistance was applied in full knee extension. The pain was more severe when kneeling on the floor. Upon examination, an abnormal protrusion was revealed in the front part of the knee that was tender when pressure was applied.

The etiology of this injury or disease is not known. It is mentioned in most texts, however, dealing with athletic injuries, that repeated blows to the front of the knee or prolonged kneeling will result in this type of injury.

General Signs and Symptoms

1. Pain and tenderness
2. Swelling
3. Pain during flexion of the knee
4. Local heat

Treatment

1. In acute stage, apply a posterior splint while knee is in full extension.

2. Ultrasound application has been proven very helpful when applied under water.

3. Application of cold packs preceding ultrasound.

Note: Osgood-Schlatter's disease usually persists for several weeks. When it becomes a chronic injury, it is best to be treated surgically.

Special Notation

In moderate to severe knee injuries the physical therapy techniques discussed here are only applicable after surgery has been considered, applied or has been ruled out.

10. Ankle Injuries and Care

General Discussion

The ankle joint is a complex hinge joint that is made up of the tibia, fibula, and talus. It is complex because it allows more movements than a typical mechanical hinge. It is a hinge joint for both the tibia and fibula and the talus, which is located underneath the tibia and fibula. The tibia and fibula form a socket (an opening or hollow that forms a holder), wider in front than behind, in which the talus moves. The ankle joint is encased with ligaments, tendons, and the synovial sheath. Major blood vessels and nerves contribute to its efficient functioning. It is a relatively small joint, but it has an important task to perform: transmitting the body weight to the foot while standing, walking, and running. Consequently, in soccer, the ankle joint is subjected to frequent violent movements, which makes it the most frequently injured joint next to the knee. (Figure 41)

There are two main movements of the ankle joint: (1) dorsiflexion, raising the foot upwards, and (2) plantar flexion, a downward motion of the foot. Any lateral movement of the ankle is not possible because of the enclosure of the talus by large bones, namely, the calcaneus, cuboid, and navicular, which, along with the three cuneiforms, form the tarsus. It is imperative to mention these bones because their movements of inversion, eversion, and circumduction, along with dorsal and plantar flexion, are the most intricate ones to a soccer player. Injury to the ankle joint occurs as a result of powerful exertion by the tendons on the bony levers. Consequently, the joint is forced beyond its normal limitation of range, resulting in temporary distortion of the foot, the leg, and the joint in between. Soft tissues are wrenched and/or torn, and blood vessels are ruptured. As adhesions occur, the muscles are contracting naturally to protect further damage, and, consequently, they immobilize the ankle.

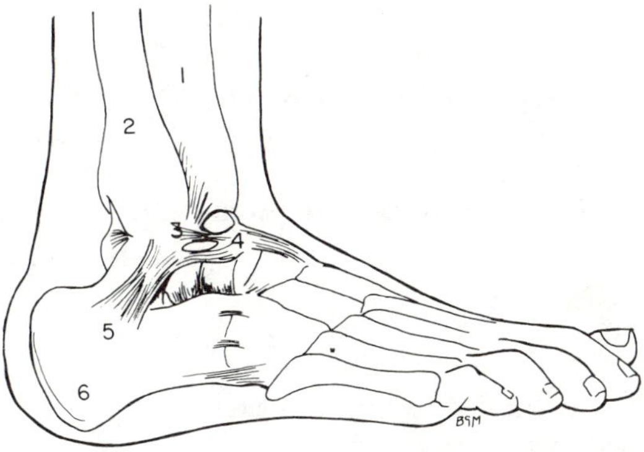

Figure 41. The Ankle Joint: 1. Tibia 2. Fibula 3, 4. Lateral Ligaments 5. Talus 6. Calcaneus

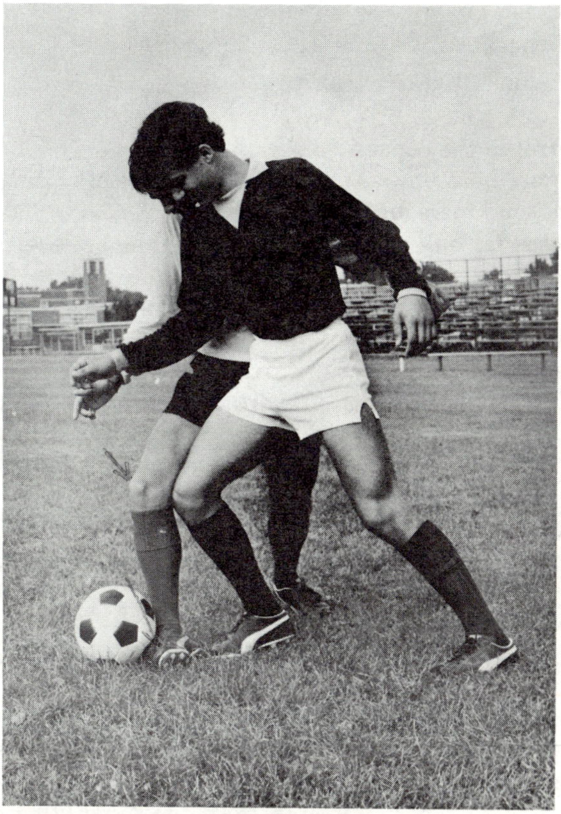

Figure 41a. Possible site of ankle and knee injury.

Signs and Symptoms

Note: Most ankle injuries occur (except direct blow or violence) to unconditioned athletes. Therefore, conditioning remains the number-one factor in injury prevention.

The most common signs and symptoms are:

1. Pain
2. Inability to place weight
3. Disability
4. Swelling
5. Immobility (lack of range of motion)
6. Increased local temperature
7. Generalized fatigue
8. Deformity

Diagnostic Tests (once X-ray has ruled out fracture)

1. Determine the cause.
2. Compare both ankles in size and in range of motion.
3. Functional tests for ankle.

a. *Dorsiflexion*—raise the foot toward the knee with gentle assistance.

b. *Plantar Flexion*—point toe downward away from the knee by providing gentle assistance.

c. *Inversion*—turn foot inward toward the midline of the body.

d. *Eversion*—turn foot outward away from the midline of the body.

e. *Circumduction*—have the foot and ankle swing freely in a circular movement around the lower leg.

The trainer's knowledge of the normal movements of the ranges of the ankle will help in diagnosing the extent of the injury of the foot and ankle.

4. Palpate for pain.

Note: The results of the evaluation should be recorded to be used as a guide for future treatment to subsequent injuries of the same part. After the initial first-aid application, the athlete should be kept mobile under physical-therapy observation; otherwise, the normal functions of the ankle will be lost. All sprains initially should be treated as fractures, and the proper splinting techniques should be applied (air splints) until the athlete has been transferred to an emergency hospital room. When the possibility of fracture has been ruled out, then proceed with the diagnostic tests and, consequently, with the rehabilitation of the ankle according to the degree of injury.

Mild Sprain

Mild ankle sprains are characterized by minimal swelling, tenderness and pain during R.O.M. (range of motion), as a result of overstretching ankle structures (ligaments) beyond their normal limitations.

First Day

1. Ethyl chloride application as described earlier.
2. Applications of ice packs while the foot is elevated above the shoulder level (athlete is lying on his back). If ice packs are not available, use regular small sponges saturated in cold water, wrapped with aluminum foil, and placed in freezer for 15 minutes.
3. Apply a flexible ace bandage in a figure-eight form as in (Figures 42a, b.)
4. Active R.O.M. should be encouraged within the tolerance of pain.
5. Use crutches in walking with non-weight bearing on injured leg.
6. Keep leg elevated during rest and on two pillows during sleep; apply ice packs if the ankle is painful, using a plastic wrap and secure them in position with an ace bandage.

Second Day

1. Whirlpool applications at temperatures of 95–96° F., with application of ultrasound at 1.2–1.5 watts/cc.[2]
2. Active R.O.M. of the ankle inside the water should be encouraged.
3. Active exercises of the other muscles of the foreleg and foot as well as the knee and hip of the injured limb should be encouraged.
4. Partial weight bearing (ball of the foot) should start per athlete's tolerance.
5. Keep leg elevated at night and proceed with active R.O.M. of the ankle and foot, emphasizing dorsiflexion, plantar flexion, inversion, eversion, and circumduction as described earlier.

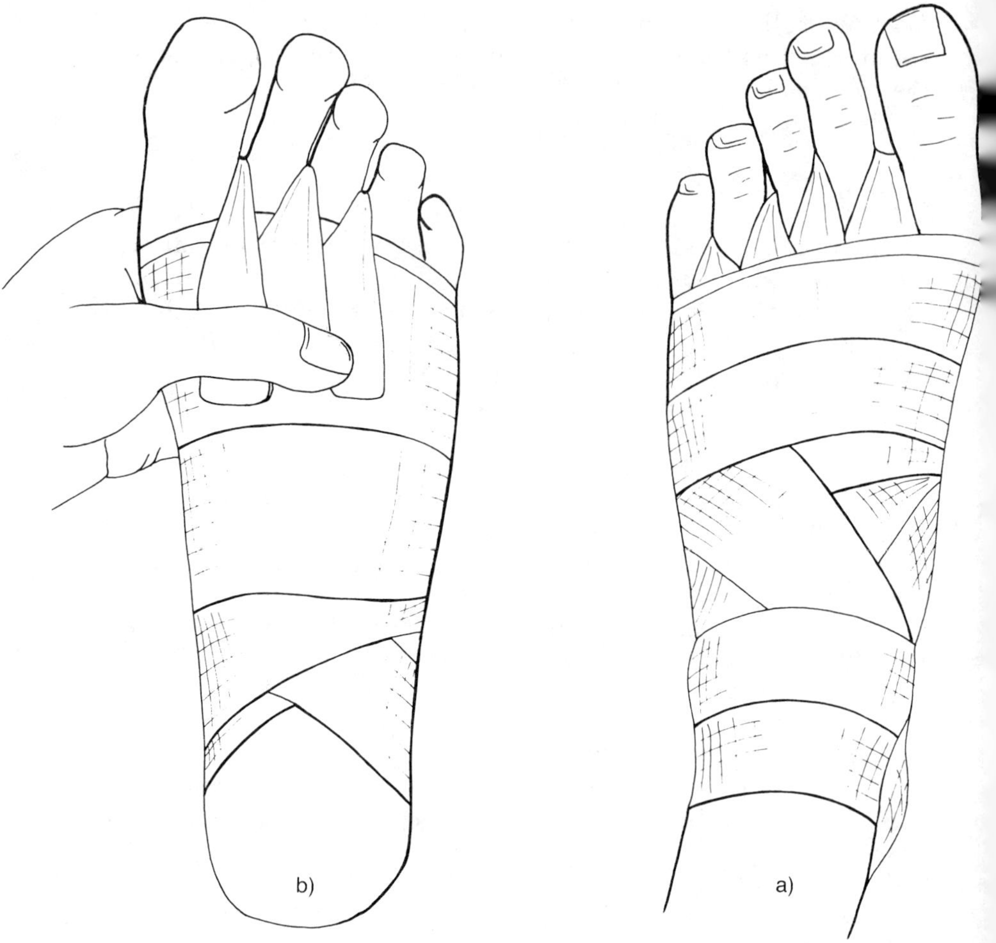

Figure 42 a, b. Application of Ace-bandage figure-eight form: a. dorsal surface; b. plantar.

Third Day

1. Whirlpool applications at 108–110° F. with active movements of the ankle inside the water.
2. Gentle soothing massage around the injured area.
3. Ultrasound application at 1.5–2.0 watts/cc.[2]
4. Active resistive exercises to all movements of ankle, foot, knee, and hip with emphasis to the former.
5. Full weight bearing with the ankle strapped with an ace bandage in figure-eight form.

6. Calisthenics, beginning with jogging and proceeding to more complicated tasks.

Fourth Day

1. Functional testing examination to determine whether full range of motion is possible. If there is absence of pain, set up a full exercise program (P.R.E. with weights or manual resistance).
2. Apply whirlpool at 108–110° F.
3. Apply elastic protective strapping.
4. Nighttime care—continue with elevation and analgesics.

Note: After active and active resistive exercises and/or a practicing session on the field, some swelling is expected. Consequently, apply a protective elastic bandage during practice and afterward.

Moderate Sprains

Moderate ankle sprains are characterized by tearing of the ligamentous fibers, moderate swelling, marked local tenderness, and considerable limitation in R.O.M. Their immediate care includes:

1. Ice packs for 48 hours.
2. Elevation.
3. Taping the ankle (close Gibney style); see earlier description and illustrations.
4. From the third day and on, whirlpool at 105–110° F., active assistive R.O.M., progressive resistive exercises.
5. In the event the ankle is immobilized, isometric exercises are encouraged within pain tolerance.

Note: On a moderate ankle sprain, I would suggest the type of splinting that can be removed for active R.O.M. to take place. The immobilization resulting from a permanent cast will prolong the rehabilitation of the ankle. For strapping demonstrations of the ankle on the third, fourth, and fifth day postinjury. (See Figure 43.) The length of disability and consequent return to the field is approximately 6–7 weeks.

Severe Complicated Sprain

In severe complicated sprains, there is considerable swelling, marked deformity, and complete loss of function. The pain is very

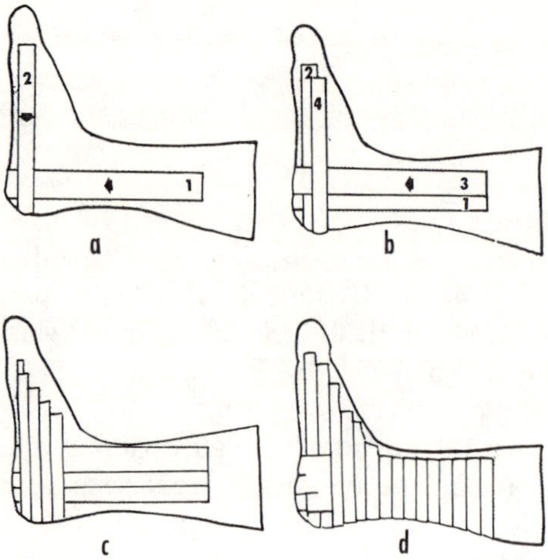

Figure 43. Demonstrating step-by-step approach of ankle strapping.

severe; in fact, athletes with severe sprain have reported more pain than those with fracture of the ankle. Surgery in many cases is the only solution to repair the torn ligaments. Short leg cast is applied, which is removed after 4–6 weeks. Rehabilitation and physical therapy begin after the cast is removed with whirlpool, ultrasound, active and active-resistive R.O.M., and, finally, progressive resistive exercise. Physical therapy is also directed to the surrounding tissues as well as those above and below the injured area, emphasizing total musculoskeletal (maintain normal R.O.M. and muscle strength) care.

Fractures of the Ankle

I will not spend much time in discussing ankle fractures because their treatment is similar to ankle sprains. The length of disability, however, is much longer, and usually the playing season for the athlete is lost. The average immobilization period is between 6 and 10 weeks, at which time the limb is in a plaster cast, extending usually from the base of the toes to the base of the patella (knee cap). During the period of immobilization, isometric exercises should be encouraged for the purpose of maintaining the muscle tone and for the prevention of muscle waste. After the cast is removed, physical-therapy techniques are applied as discussed in ankle sprains.

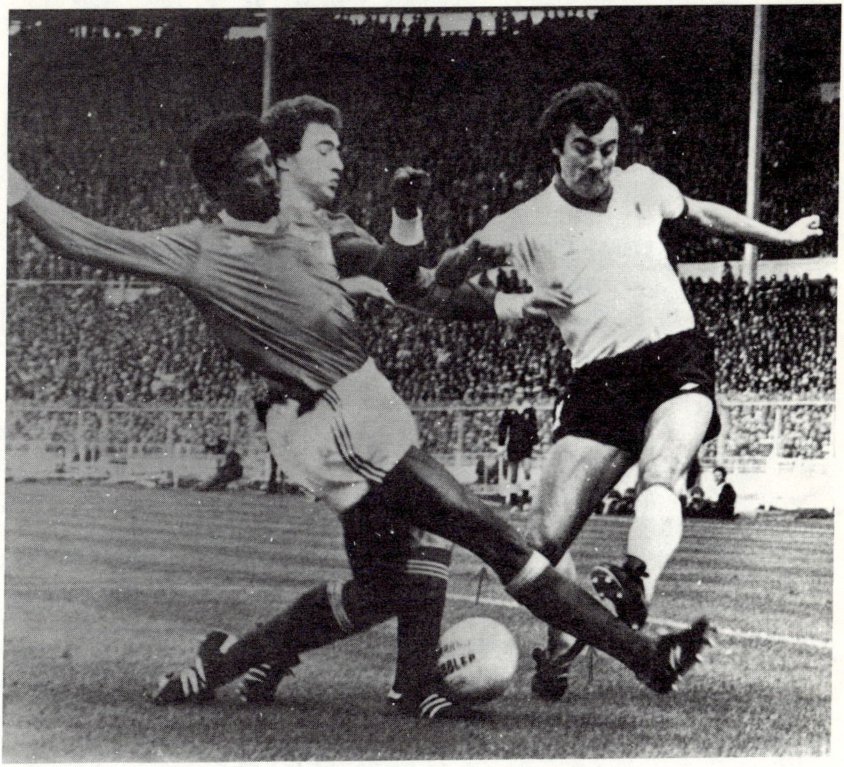

Figure 43a. Arrows, pointing to sites of injury, knee and ankle.

Most Common Sites of Sprains

The most common sites of ankle sprains occur on the lateral border of the ankle. (Figure 44) The lateral border (outside border of the ankle) is injured at a ratio of 10 to 1 as compared to the medial border. Therefore, medial ligament injuries are very rare. When they do occur, however, similar techniques are applied. Their length of recovery, however, is longer because they respond to treatment much more slowly than the lateral ligaments. Consequently, athletes with arch problems of prolonged periods are the ones mostly injured on the medial border. To prevent such injuries from recurring, caused by fallen arches, arch supports, ¼ inch lift inside the heel, and progressive resistive exercises to gastrosoleus and tibialis anterior groups are strongly advocated.

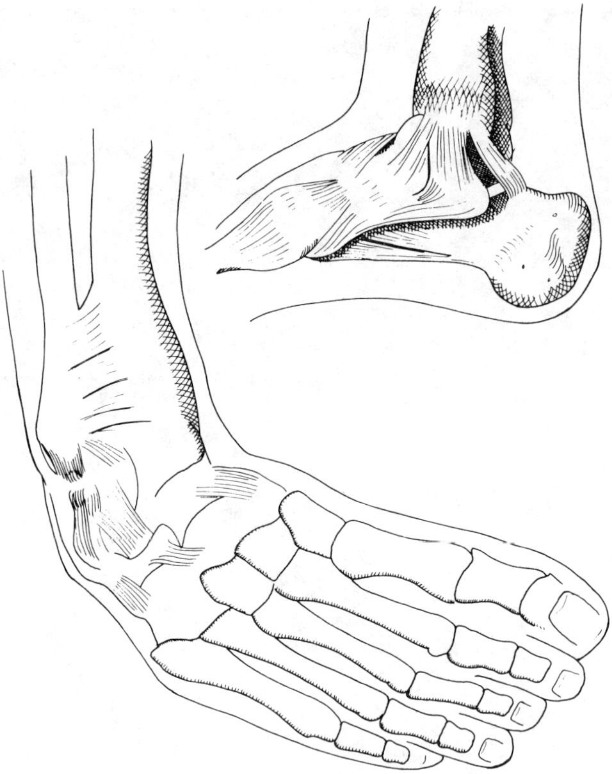

Figure 44. Ruptured lateral ligaments of the ankle after a severe sprain.

Ankle Strains

Ankle strains occur as such in ankle injuries or in combination with ankle sprains. The term *strain*, also known as "muscle pull," is a condition that is brought about by forcing the muscle to go beyond its expected range when subjected to the stress of uncoordinated action. Consequently, the muscle will be either torn completely or partially. The degree of involvement will depend on the number of torn fibers. If the injury is severe enough to cause additional damage to the ligaments, then it will be diagnosed as a sprain. Technically, therefore, we might say that a mild muscle pull is a strain where a more severe one will be a sprain. The treatment that follows, therefore, will be similar to that of sprain and will be treated accordingly: mild, moderate, or severe.

Immediate Care After Injury

1. Compression ace bandage preimmersed in water or flexible adhesive cast.
2. Ice-pack application on the injured area to be secured by another elastic bandage.
3. Elevation.
4. Weight bearing should be partial or eliminated.

Second Day

1. Whirlpool baths at 96–98-dg F.
2. Electrical currents with mild intensity
3. Gentle active R.O.M.
4. Partial weight bearing to tolerance

Third Day

1. Whirlpool baths at 105–110° F. with active R.O.M. of the ankle while inside the whirlpool
2. Active-resistive R.O.M.
3. Ultrasound at 1.5 watts/cc^2 on the injured area and along a 4–6-inch radius
4. Elastic bandage during walking hours and during rest if tolerable
5. Calisthenics (slow stretching) and field activities by the end of the week

Note: The length of disability of muscle pulls in their mild form is less than their respective ankle sprains.

The speed with which an athlete recovers from an ankle injury will depend on the immediate first-aid procedures and the rehabilitation techniques used to restore normal function to the ankle. The knowledge of the anatomy and physiology of the human body in evaluating and, consequently, applying the most appropriate modalities and exercise programs are the major tools in providing the care that results in normal functioning. The misuse of modalities or the early application of exercises and weight bearing after ankle injuries could be detrimental to an early recovery and, consequently, the result of a chronically painful and disabled ankle.

Of course, if the athlete has been attending training regularly, participating in precondition exercises and warmups, such preventive measures will not only limit the number of injuries but enable him to recover from the injury within a shorter period of time.

11. Thigh Injuries and Care

General Discussion

The thigh contains the longest and strongest bone of the body, the femur (Figure 45). The femur is composed of two parts, the upper part, which connects to the hip joint and, consequently, the acetabulum of the pelvis; the lower part, which connects to the knee joint and, consequently, the tibia, the figula, and the patella. The muscles of the thigh are divided into groups whose primary functions are directly related to their anatomic position or to the place where each muscle is situated. For example, when the muscles inside the thigh known as adductors contract, they bring the thigh inward. The muscles on the outside of the thigh during contraction bring the thigh outward. The front muscles flex the hip by bringing the thigh upward, and the back

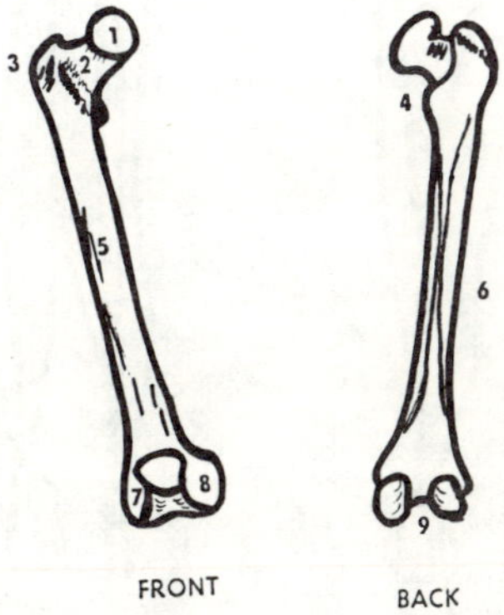

Figure 45. Front and back view of the femur. (1) Head of femur. (2) Neck of femur. (3) Greater trochanter. (4) Lesser trochanter. (5) Shaft of femur. (6) Linca aspera. (7) Lateral condyle. (8) Medial condyle. (9) Intercondylar notch.

muscles extend the hip by bringing the thigh backward (Figures 46a, b). More complicated movements as those in internal (inward) and external (outward) rotations, which occur, with very few exceptions, according to the anatomic position of the muscles. Most of the injuries with which I have been involved were limited to three major groups, specifically, the quadriceps, the hamstrings, and the muscles of the groin or the adductor and iliopsoas groups. The quadriceps' main function is to extend the knee joint; it covers most of the front of the thigh. The hamstrings' main function is to flex the knee joint and is located on the back of the thigh. The adductors of the thigh are located on the inside of the thigh. The most frequent injuries to the thigh are limited to muscle contusions, muscle pulls, and ruptured muscles, partially or completely. The most common sites of injury to the thigh are: (1) hamstrings (semitendinosis, semimembranosus, biceps femoris) and (2) quadriceps (rectus femoris). Damage to the thigh muscles may take place at the upper end, known as the origin, or at their lower end near the knee joint, known as the insertion, or at the center of their muscle bulk, known as the belly of the muscle. The condition may involve a

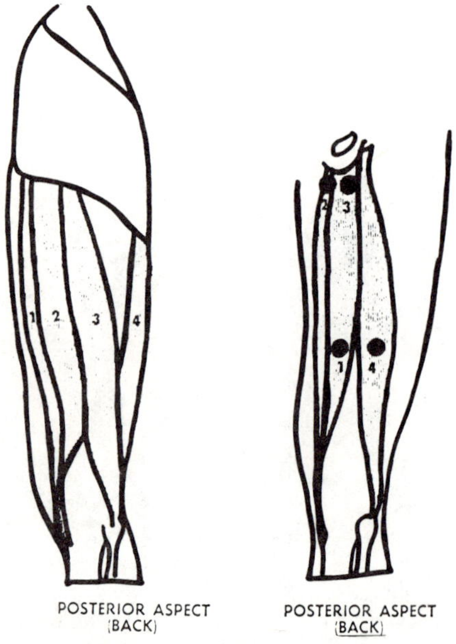

Figure 46a. Posterior muscles: 1. Semimembranosus; 2. Semitendinonos; 3. Biceps Femorus; 4. Vastus Lateralis; 5. Most common sites of injury.

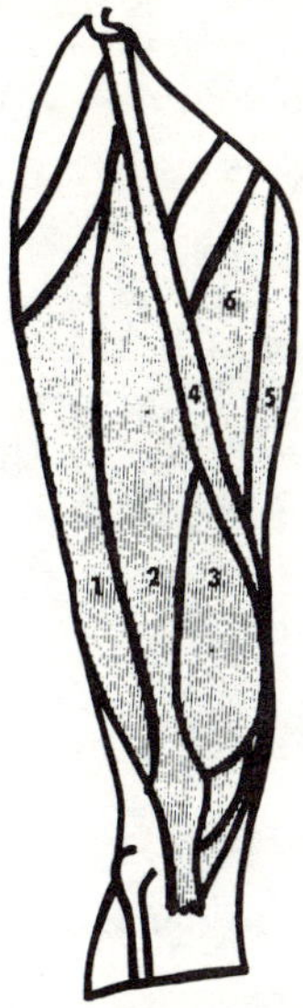

Figure 46b. Anterior (front) muscles of the thigh. 1. Vastus lateralis; 2. Rectus femoris; 3. Vastus medialis; 4. Sartorius; 5. Gracilias; 6. Adductor longus.

few muscle fibers or complete tearing of the muscle. The degree of limitation and consequent disability is dependent on the number of muscle fibers torn, the amount of hemorrhage, and the formation of thick adhesions. Consequently, the correct first aid immediately administered reduces greatly the hemorrhage as well as the formation of thick adhesions.

Signs and Symptoms

Whether a few or many fibers are involved or even a complete tear of a muscle, the signs and symptoms are approximately the same except that they differ in the degree of limitation of movement and pain, both excellent diagnostic signs and indicators of the therapeutic procedures to be applied. The signs and symptoms are:

1. Sudden splitting pain
2. Local tenderness
3. Athlete can't move extremity (limb)
4. Muscle spasm

5. Limited passive and active movement
6. Stiffness
7. Often feels the muscle is "broken"
8. Discoloration
9. Swelling
10. Occasionally non-weight bearing

Note: The etiology, which I have repeatedly mentioned, is the unpreparedness of the athlete from either lack of warmup or not enough warmup. Under this condition, any sudden twisting or unprepared muscle contraction will result in an injury. A direct blow to the front or back of the thigh will also result in an injury.

Contusions

A thigh contusion is an injury in which muscle tissues are broken—usually from a direct blow—while the overlying area of the skin remains unbroken. In a muscle pull, however, the pain is acquired due to the pulling or tear of muscle fibers, resulting not from a direct blow but from the act of running and/or sudden take off. A contusion is also known by many athletes as a charley horse. The differentiating diagnosis is very important for the treatment that will follow. Therefore, a charley horse should be related to a trauma resulting from a blow received and will be also known as contusion, while a muscle pull is related to sudden pain that occurred in the process of running. Thus, during a blow to the front of the thigh, the contused muscles are painful during flexion of the knee; while a blow to the back muscles of the thigh will result in pain when the knee is extended.

Mild Contusion, Anterior (front) or Posterior Back Thigh Muscles

1. First 24 hours: check for limitation in R.O.M. (Figure 47) to determine degree of injury.
2. Apply an elastic compression bandage either 4 inches or 6 inches in width soaked into water.
3. Apply cold packs on the injured part and its surrounded tissues.
4. Secure cold packs with another elastic (dry) bandage 4 inches or 6 inches in width.
5. Keep leg elevated.

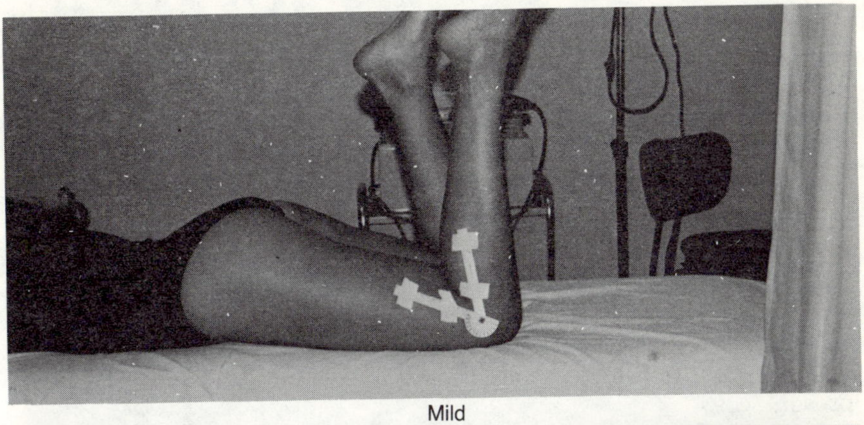

Mild

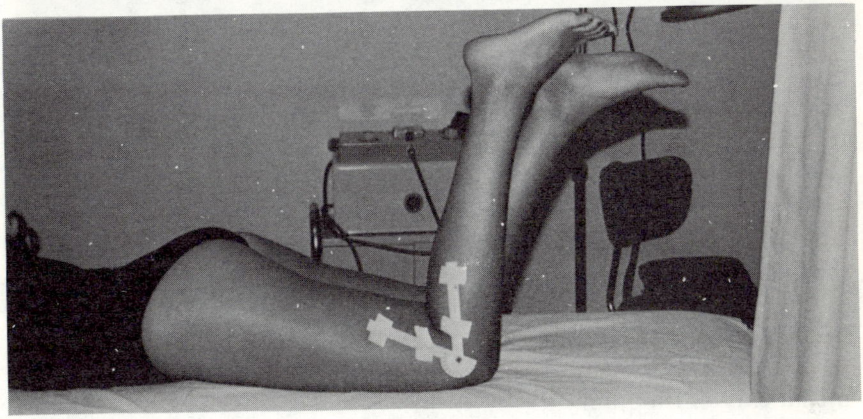

Moderate

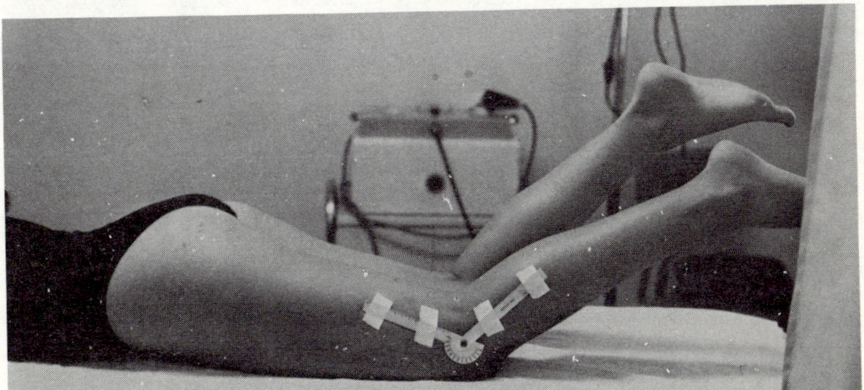

Severe

Figure 47. Photographic interpretation of anterior thigh contusion as athlete lies on abdomen.

After 24 hours or second day of injury

1. Check limitation in R.O.M. (range of motion) of the knee joint, flexion or extension.

2. Application of heat (whirlpool at 104–108° F.), for approximately 30 minutes.

3. Active exercises inside whirlpool, flexing or extending the knee joint.

4. Lying prone/supine (quadriceps and hamstrings, respectively) on a treatment table, flex the knee or extend slowly for many repetitions.

5. Apply to number 4 mild resistance when very minimum pain present.

Note: When the quadriceps are injured, apply resistance initially in flexion by resisting the hamstrings. This procedure will relax the quadriceps. Then proceed with mild resistance to the quadriceps. Repeat the same procedure, but in reverse, when the hamstrings are injured. This phenomenon is known as *reciprocal innervation* or reverse of antagonists. It is a phenomenon that can be very helpful when it is fully understood.

6. Apply contrast (heat and cold) application upon completion of the exercise at 5-minute intervals.

Special Notation: The length of an athlete's disability will depend on the athlete's physiological response to his injury as well as the athlete's initial care of the injury.

After the Third Day

1. Application of heat (whirlpool or hydrocollator hot packs)
2. Application of ultrasonic within the water
3. Manual resistive exercises
4. Progressive resistive exercises (De Lorme method)
5. Application of elastic adhesive before practice and games (Figure 48)

Moderate to Severe Contusions

First 48 hours:

1. Compression with elastic adhesive tape.

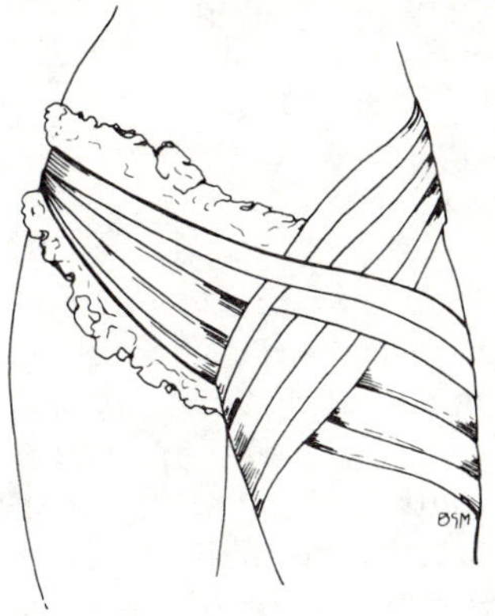

Figure 48. Application of elastic self-adhesive compression bandage extending from mid-thigh and anchored at the waist. Pretaping material is necessary.

2. Ice-pack application.
3. Elevation of the extremity and rest.
4. Keep knee in flexion between 15–25° F (it helps to reduce pain on hamstrings).
5. Strapping must start below the knee and proceed all the way up to the thigh. (Some of the thigh muscles are situated below the knee.) Use a 4-inch adhesive elastic bandage.
6. No weight bearing is allowed at this time.

Third Day

1. Continue ice packs until pain disappears or is considerably minimized.
2. Check R.O.M. of the knee joint.
3. When the pain and discomfort during movement have been minimized considerably, apply hydrocollator hot packs on the anterior and posterior surfaces.
4. Heat should be applied after the compression adhesive bandage has been removed—apply moist heat for 30 minutes.
5. Massage above and below the contused area—not on the top—mildly (efflaurage).
6. Proceed the next day with ultrasonic application progressively from 1.0 to 1.75 watts/cc.[2]
7. Begin active R.O.M. exercises to pain tolerance until full R.O.M. is accomplished.
8. Once full R.O.M. is accomplished in flexion and extension of

the knee joint, proceed with manual resistive exercise, applying the reciprocal innervation phenomenon as described in the previous pages.

9. When considerable manual resistance is tolerable, proceed with progressive resistance exercises in the N/K table (quadriceps table with weights).

Special Note: This disability may last between two and six weeks, depending on the degree and number of damaged muscle fibers, the initial care, and the continuation of such care. A severe contusion, as determined by Figure 47, will take approximately 6–8 weeks before the player can participate in field workout. When the player begins his participation, he must have his leg strapped with an elastic self-adhesive ace bandage as illustrated previously.

Ruptured Adductor (Groin)

Groin injuries are the other most common injuries occurring to the soccer athlete in poor physical condition because his muscles cannot tolerate sudden pulls and cannot generally withstand strain. Groin injuries occur during a sideward movement or a split of both legs either sideways or forwards. If the injury occurs during a forward split, the injured muscle is the iliopsoas, the muscle responsible for kicking the ball in cooperation with the quadriceps. If the injury occurs during a sideward split, the injured muscle is the adductor, the muscle responsible in keeping the thighs together. The aftercare of both injuries is the same.

Immediate Treatment

Compression bandage (the self-adhesive type) extending from the mid-thigh and anchored at the waist several times as in Figure 49.

Special Note: In view of the anatomic situation of the injury, the application of ice is very difficult; consequently, the best first aid will be the compression bandage followed by rest. Avoid as much weight bearing on the injured leg as possible, and use crutches if necessary.

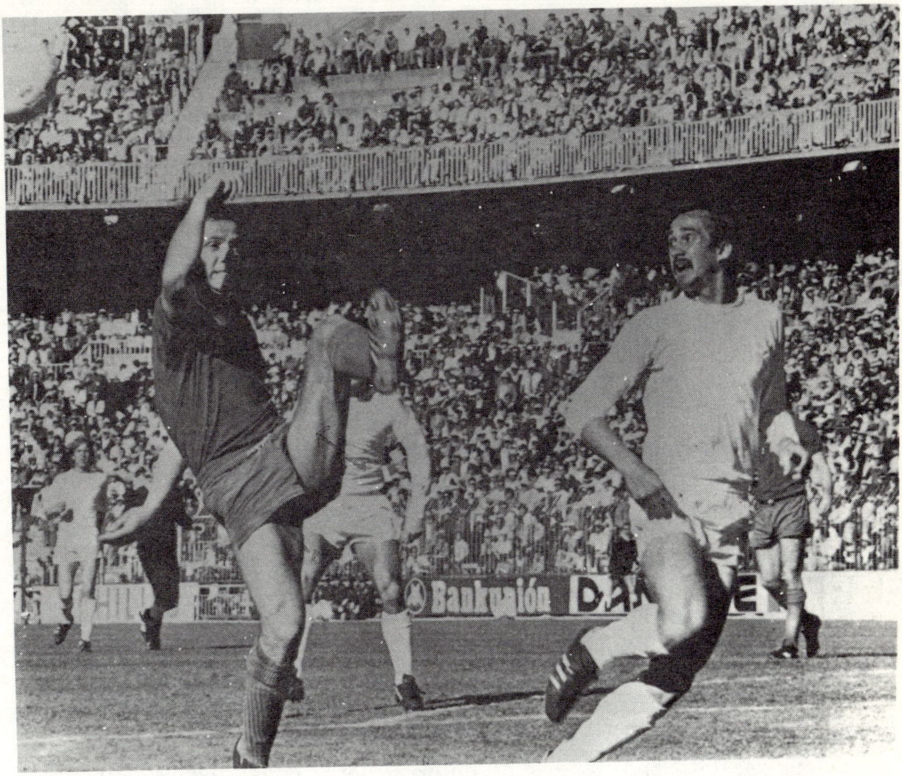

Figure 49a. Possible sites of pulled muscles: and/or ruptured a) groin, b) hamstring.

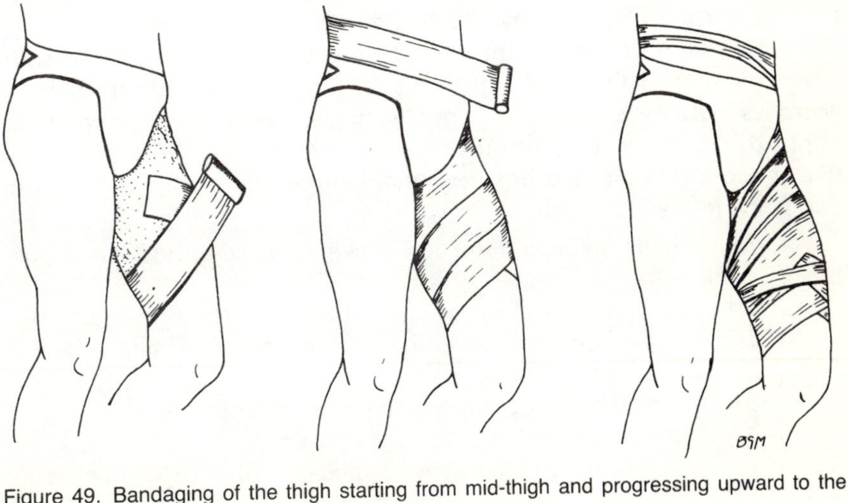

Figure 49. Bandaging of the thigh starting from mid-thigh and progressing upward to the waist for anchorage with flexible elastic strap.

After the Second Day

1. Whirlpool at 108° F. with mild active movement to pain tolerance.

2. Ultrasonic between 1.5 and 1.75 watts/cc.^{2} over the painful area and over the lumbo sacral area.

3. Active R.O.M., emphasizing abduction and flexion of the hip, mildly.

4. When pain, discomfort, and full abduction and flexion of the hip are attained, proceed with manual resistive exercises or use sandbag weights with velcro closures.

5. During practice sessions or games, apply elastic self-adhesive cast as in Figure 49.

Note: Disability may last between 2 and 4 weeks. Proper care with exercise and preventive measures will reduce the time of disability.

Myositis Ossificans

Myositis Ossificans is an inflammation of muscle fibers with thick formation of adhesions that turn into calcifications. It starts usually as a severe contusion—mostly at the front muscles of the thigh—of the quadriceps, which either does not respond to treatment or is being mistreated during its initial state. When after two–three weeks the quadriceps fail to show signs of improvement, it is suspected that myositis ossificans has occurred. This muscular calcified mass on the quadricep muscle becomes a handicap to the athlete. Flexion and extension of the knee joint are limited, and recurrent blows, in view of the proximity of the thigh, increase the disability. The treatment that follows may vary from the application of hip spica and ambulation on crutches with non-weight bearing to more liberal methods of heat applications using such modalities as ultrasound and diathermy. The use of the latter method has been more successful in my experience, using the following routine:

1. Moist heat (hydrocollator hot packs) on both anterior and posterior surfaces for 30 minutes.

2. Ultrasound applications at 1.2–1.8 watts/cc.^{2} for 6 to 8 minutes.

3. Isometric exercises progressively increasing in time (6–15 seconds) of muscular contractions, 10 repetitions.

4. Mild to moderate massage (efflaurage to petrissage).

5. Mild passive movements to pain tolerance.

6. An elastic bandage should be applied—as illustrated in charley

horse—when the patient is placing weight on injured leg.

Special Notations

1. The above treatment should be applied daily.
2. Rest must be emphasized, and only minimal activity should be allowed.
3. The athlete is removed from all field activity.
4. Complete absorption of the calcified muscle mass might take from 3 to 6 months.
5. Surgical procedure for removal of calcium is seldom indicated.

Quadriceps Pull

Muscle pull is also known as muscle strain; therefore, when we discuss pulled muscles, we will also be discussing strained muscles. Poor condition and improper warmup are also the predisposing factors. A quadriceps pull means that the muscle fibers (few, many, or total tear) have been forced to go beyond their normal limitation. The degree of injury and consequent disability is dependent on the number of muscle fibers that have been damaged. In soccer injuries, a complete tear is very seldom seen but should not be overlooked during our initial evaluation.

First 24–48 hours

1. Apply ethyl chloride on suspected muscle pull (method of application has been discussed in the previous chapter) at the approximate point of the injury.
2. Apply a wet elastic bandage, 4–6 inches in width, extending from just above the knee cap to the upper three-quarters of the thigh.
3. Ice-pack application over the wet ace bandage.
4. Secure ice pack with another ace bandage.
5. Rest and elevation of the limb should follow.

After 24–48 hours

1. Whirlpool at 108° F. after 48 hours for moderate or severe in-

jury. Keep the turbines, which cause the turbulence, away from the injured part.

2. Ultrasonic waves, 1.5–2.0 watts/cc.[2]

3. Electrical currents, pulse rate muscle contraction (approximately 10 minutes).

4. Massage to be applied mildly as in milking the quadriceps.

5. Active exercises of the quadriceps from the supine position with straight leg raising for 6 counts.

6. Manual resistive exercises from semilying position.

7. Progressive resistive exercise begins after full R.O.M. inflexion and extension has been attained.

8. Stretching exercises with caution to both quadriceps and hamstrings.

a. stretching quadriceps—lying prone (on stomach), reach back and grasp the ankle and hold—*do not pull suddenly and sharply*.

b. stretching hamstrings—semilying position, spread legs appart (18–24 inches) and attempt to touch toes without bending knees.

9. Mild workout with the thigh strapped as in Figure 49. Normal walking, fast walking, jogging, and sprinting should be the progression of the workout on the field.

10. After the field workout, remove strapping, apply contrast heat and cold packs (5-minute intervals) and mild stretching. Then strap thigh again.

Ruptured Quadriceps

The muscle most likely to rupture from the anterior muscles of the thigh is the rectus femoris. The reason for this is that the rectus femoris connects two joints involved in flexing the hip and extending the knee, respectively. Therefore, its length as well as its anatomic proximity—directly in front of the thigh—increase its susceptibility to injury. A ruptured rectus femoris means that there is a break in its continuity leading to loss of function and consequent disability. Inadequate warmup to prepare its strength as well as inadequate stretching for the preparation of its flexibility are the leading causes of this injury. Additional causes are: (1) knee bends and squatting too early in the season, (2) returning to field activity too soon after having a fracture cast, (3) hypertrophy of the quadriceps without adequate antagonism of the hamstrings, (4) existing myositis ossificans while engaged in activity.

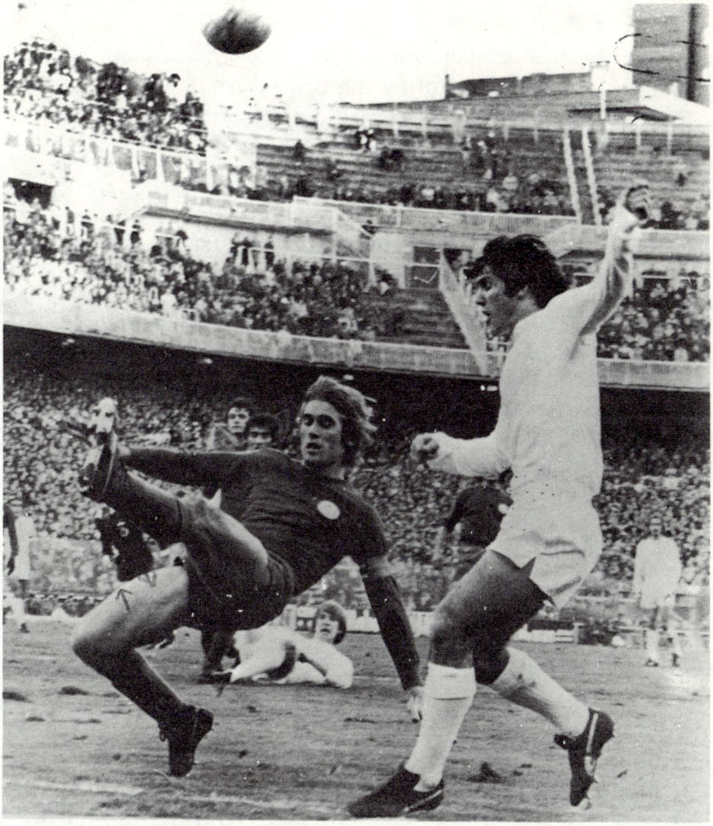

Figure 50a. Possible rupture of quadriceps.

Signs and Symptoms

1. Functional loss.
   a. Leg can not be extended fully.
   b. Walking with limp.
2. Knee cap drops slightly downward.
3. Pain upon weight bearing and/or during flexion and extension of the knee joint.
4. Crepitations present during muscle contractions.
5. Swelling above and below the tear.

Treatment

When the tear is not complete, and surgery has been ruled out by the orthopedic surgeon, the following procedure should be applied:

1. Flexible cast with knee in full extension (Figure 50).
2. Ice pack applications for 48 hours.
3. Night splint, maintaining knee in full extension.
4. Whirlpool daily (after 48 hours) at 105° F.
5. Electrical stimulation with pulsating current.
6. Mild active assistive R.O.M. to be followed with active R.O.M.
7. Mild resistive exercise when full R.O.M. in flexion and extension of the knee joint has been attained.
8. Progressive resistive exercise when healing is complete and pain is absent.
9. Field workouts same as in previous procedure.
10. Flexible cast should be applied in all workouts.

Special Notations: Muscle atrophy should be prevented at any cost. Isometric exercises should be emphasized within the flexible cast.

Ruptured Hamstrings

The causes resulting in rupturing the hamstrings are the same ones outlined for ruptured rectus femoris. Any break in the continuity of biceps femoris, semitendinosis, and semimembranosus will result in a ruptured hamstring and will lead to partial temporary disability

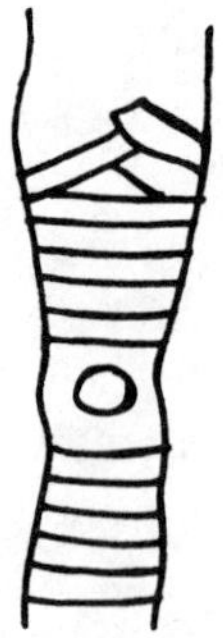

Figure 50. Ruptured quadriceps in flexible cast. Flexible cast with knee in full extension during ruptured quadriceps.

of the athlete. Prevention through the proper stretching and strengthening exercises will be the best therapy.

Signs and Symptoms

1. Severe pain upon weight bearing.
2. Swelling above and below the tear.
3. Localized tenderness.
4. Discoloration.
5. A concavity at the break of the muscle easily palpable.
6. The athlete will have difficulty flexing or extending his knee because of the pain and stiffness.

Treatment

When the tear is not complete, and surgery has been ruled out, the treatment that will follow will be similar to the one applied to ruptured rectus femoris. The flexible cast will be applied with the knee flexed to approximately 20–25°. (Figure 51) The flexible cast can be removed after the third day for heat applications and exercises as described previously. The flexible cast should be reapplied after every treatment session. Every effort should be made to keep the athletes as active as possible even with the flexible casts in order to prevent atrophy of these muscles.

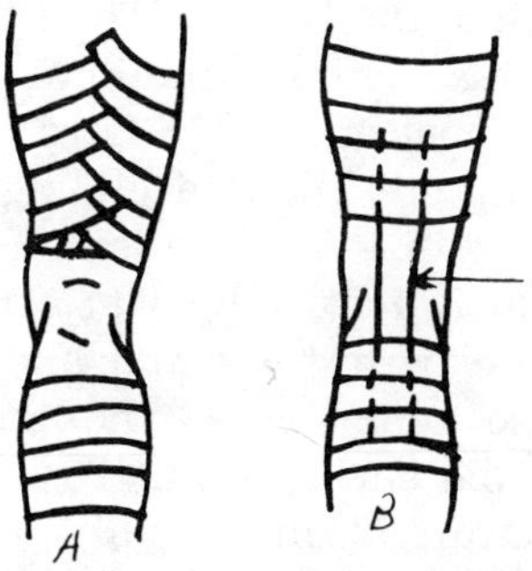

Figure 51. Ruptured hamstrings in flexible cast. Flexible cast to rupture hamstrings with the knee flexed at 25 degrees. Orthoplast material to keep knee flexed is indicated by the arrow.

12. Lower Leg Injuries and Care

General Discussion

Injuries to the knee joint as well as injuries to the ankle joint have been discussed in earlier chapters. Injuries to the lower leg involve the muscles and bones between the knee and the ankle.

The muscles of the lower leg are divided into three groups and are situated anteriorly, posteriorly, and laterally. Their anatomic positions—the same as those of the thigh muscles—determine the course of their action on the lower part of the leg. Thus, the posterior muscles operate during contraction to plantar—flex the ankle (forcing the toes to point downward or, during standing, forcing toe standing); the anterior muscles operate during contraction to dorsiflex the ankle (forcing toes upward closer to the shin bone or standing on heels), and the lateral muscles operate during contraction, forcing the foot to bear weight on the instep.

Of the muscles of the lower leg, only one muscle crosses the knee joint, and two muscles cross both the knee and ankle joints. It is worthwhile to mention this fact because injury to one of these muscles will limit the normal function of both joints. (Figure 52)

The tibia and fibula, the bones of the lower leg, have been mentioned earlier (in the discussion of the knee and ankle injuries). The slender fibula, on its upper end, articulates with the tibia, forming a synovial joint (allowing only limited gliding movement), and on its lower end articulates with the lateral side (outside the ankle joint). The tibia, or shin bone, is a much heavier bone of the lower leg; at its upper end, it articulates with the femur and fibula; at its lower end, it articulates with the talar bone of the ankle and the tibia fibula syndesmosis (no articular surfaces, only ligaments).

Injuries in the nature of muscle pulls, contusions, and ruptured muscles of the lower leg are quite common among soccer players. Fractures of the tibia do occur in soccer, although not very often. Fractures

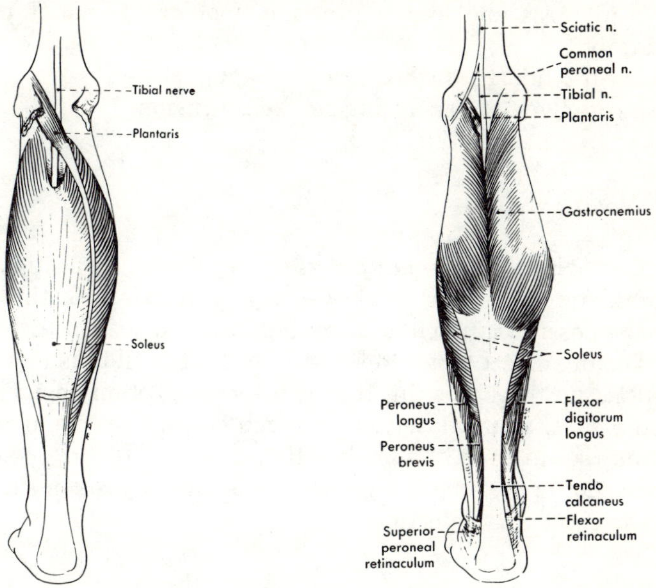

Figure 52. Superficial and deep muscles of the back of the leg.

of the tibia may occur as in associated fractures of the fibula, although they occur mainly as individual fractures to the fibula on a ratio of 2 to 1.

Signs and Symptoms

In most of the injuries, the signs and symptoms will determine the diagnosis and, consequently, the first-aid application. Careful inspection of the lower leg is very essential in arriving at the proper application of the first aid. Any severe sprain or contusion should be treated as a fracture, and the athlete should immediately be taken to the hospital for x-rays. The general signs and symptoms of mild to severe injuries to the lower leg are:

1. Tightness in the back or the front of the leg.
2. Something "popping out" in the front or the back.
3. Superficial soreness right under the skin.
4. Swelling present on the upper part of the calf muscles or the tibialis anterior, depending on the site of the injury.
5. Pain present during dorsiflexion or plantar flexion of the ankle and/or knee flexion and extension.

6. Numbness and loss of function (foot drop)—notify physician immediately.

7. Local tenderness when pressure applied.

8. Large hematomas during severe contusions.

Special Notations

1. *Do not massage or manipulate* the leg during inspection of above symptoms. According to Dr. J. V. Cerney, "any external stimulus may lead to the possibility of circulatory collapse and possible death."

2. During direct blows to the shin bone, the tibia is marked with abraded tissue (broken skin) that can form infection easily unless it is taken care of immediately. It is much easier to prevent infections before they set in than it is to alter them.

3. Do not apply any analgesics or vaseline to broken skin; it will encourage secondary infection.

Fractures of Lower Leg

Fractures along the upper border of the tibia (any of the condyles or both), will cause considerable swelling of the knee joint, considerable pain, and, consequently, loss of function. Fractures along the shaft of the tibia—mostly the lower one-third—are usually caused by direct blow. The tibia may be palpated, and even mild movement will be extremely painful, especially dorsiflexion or plantarflexion. The most common site of fracture of the fibula is the lower one-third, which may be associated with a fracture of the tibia. Pain and tenderness will be quite evident and will be more so upon movement of the ankle joint. The fibula is a non-weight bearing bone of the lower leg. The athlete may be able to walk as long as the tibia carries all the weight.

Immediate Care

1. Application of air splints and into hospital emergency care.

2. During fibula fractures, elastic compression bandage and crutches before the athlete is transported to emergency hospital care.

Note: In fractures of the lower leg, sufficient healing occurs between 4 weeks and 3 months before weight bearing is allowed. In fractures of the lower one-third of the fibula, participation or use of the soccer field is permitted after sufficient rehabilitation has taken place, resulting in normal range of motion and muscle strength. It takes usually between 4 and 6 weeks. Physical therapy modalities are quite popular and effective and are applied in the form of whirlpool, hydrocollator hot packs, ultrasound, electrical stimulation, short-wave diathermy, and last but not least, therapeutic exercise, all of which must be applied under the direct supervision of a physical therapist for maximum results in the shortest period of time.

Strains of the Lower Leg

Strains of the lower leg are obviously much more common than fractures in soccer injuries. Let me point out again that in well-trained athletes, muscle strains or muscle pulls very rarely occur. The most common site of muscle strain is seen in the posterior aspect (back) of the leg. The muscles most commonly injured are the gastrocnemius and the plantaris. Upon inspection, the athlete will reveal that he felt a "popping" sensation on the back of his leg followed by soreness upon pressure, pain, and limitation of movement, forcing the athlete to leave the field. Swelling and tightness will be apparent after palpating the group of muscles. The most common locations in order of occurrence are the medial head of the gastrocnemius (located inside the knee joint at the medial femoral tubercle), the belly of the muscles, the lateral head, and the attachment with the Achilles tendon.

Muscle strain to the plantaris muscle may be associated with injury to the Achilles tendon. It is a long slender muscle that is similar to the gastrocnemius. It is a two-joint muscle at the knee and at the ankle. Consequently, its injury affects the range of motion of both joints. Its main function is to plantar flex the ankle. When injured, the athlete will describe it as "something giving away" with considerable pain and often a snap that will be quite audible.

Immediate care for the gastrocnemius and the plantaris muscles will be the classical application of ice pack, compression with an elastic bandage, and rest. Do not apply any weight on the injured foot for at least 24–48 hours, depending on its severity as determined by the ankle and knee movements. The application of such modalities as whirlpool at 104° F., hot packs, and electrical stimulation under professional supervision, as well as therapeutic exercise, will enhance the healing process. Elastic wrappings will be very helpful and should be applied regularly after the completion of the daily treatment. After normal active range of motion has been attained, slow stretching, emphasizing dorsiflexion, should be attempted before each practice session to avoid recurrence of the injury. A soft rubber cushion ½-inch thickness placed under the heel or inside the shoe will ease the amount of muscle tension. Muscle strengthening exercises of the gastrocnemius and plantaris muscle should begin immediately after normal R.O.M. has been attained. Daily exercises in standing and walking, progressively increased to jumping on the toes with knees straight, will bring normal strength to the muscles.

The soleus muscle of the lower leg is rarely injured in soccer mostly because its action occurs in one joint, the ankle only. When it becomes injured, however, its immediate care will be the same as well as the aftercare. To test and increase its strength, however, you can apply the same exercises as those applied in the gastrocnemius, the only difference being, instead of walking and jumping on the toes with knees straight, you do the same with knees bent. Any muscle pull of the above-mentioned muscles should take between 3 and 6 weeks before the injured athlete is completely rehabilitated. If immediate care as well as aftercare is applied as outlined, under professional supervision, the degree of disability will be undoubtedly minimized, and the athlete will be able to participate actively much sooner.

Contusions of Lower Leg

Muscle contusions next to the thigh, are more likely to occur in the lower leg, especially the anterior (front) part. Any direct blow to the leg that involves the bony tissue beneath the muscle will result in the releasing of bone cells and minerals into the muscle, thereby creating a muscle contusion. If the resulting hemorrhage is not absorbed and eventually becomes ossified, the bonelike formation in the muscle is known as myositis ossificans (discussed in an earlier chapter). The most common site of muscle contusions is the anterior (front) part of the lower leg. Usually, after receiving such an injury, the athlete is able to continue the game. However, after the game, he will suffer a lot of pain and discomfort. Maximum healing of contusions can be achieved by minimizing or absorbing the formation of hematoma with ice-pack applications, compression bandage, and elevation for 24–48 hours. After immediate care, physical therapy should begin in the form of heat application—mostly moist heat and whirlpool at 105–108° F. Gentle active exercise should follow to dissolve the formation of hematomas. In contusions of deep muscles, the application of Medcosonlator is an effective modality for quickly reducing the amount of disability and enhancing normal function. When the athlete is able to return to the field (3 days for mild contusion to 3 weeks in severe contusion), effective padding and flexible casting are very essential to prevent recurring injury. Contusions, to the posterior (back) area of the lower leg and calf, are not too common. They are, however, just as disabling and painful. The most common site of contusion is the belly of the gastrocnemius and the tibialis posterior. The bleeding and, consequently, the formation of hematoma over a large area are evident. Immediate care should focus on controlling the hemorrhage with the application of ice, compression bandage, and elevation. This procedure should continue for at least 48 hours while the athlete is on bed rest—in severe contusion—and/or on crutches with non-weight bearing. After 48 hours, the physical-therapy procedure should be the same as described for the anterior area of the leg. In a mild contusion, the time of disability may extend to 2 days, while in a severe contusion the time of disability may extend to 4 weeks. However, fast recovery depends on the athlete's cooperation in following instructions and his physiological healing process.

Contusions of the tendons are not too frequent in soccer injuries. In fact, in my 15 years of treating soccer injuries, I have only once treated a lower leg contusion of the Achilles tendon. Treatment of tendon contusions is essentially the same as for muscle contusions. In the contusion of the Achilles tendon, the disability is prolonged and extended to approximately 10 weeks before the athlete's participation in the rehabilitation of these injuries both in terms of immediate care and aftercare.

Tibialis Anterior Syndrome

Tibialis anterior syndrome refers to the acute swelling occurring at the anterior (front) area of the lower leg, which results after prolonged and vigorous exercise. Considerable pain and paresis (very weak, incomplete paralysis) of the muscle follows.

Signs and Symptoms

1. Considerable swelling anteriorly.
2. Tenderness.
3. Considerable pain in attempting to lift toes and ankle along the tibial shaft.

4. Incomplete paralysis.
5. The muscle becomes very hard.
6. Partial loss of sensation of foot and toes.
7. Drop foot (athlete unable to dorsiflex the ankle).

Treatment

Once you recognize the problem, get the athlete to the hospital for emergency care.

Note: Do not attempt to move the leg or manipulate the ankle.

Charley Horse

This condition is used to describe any injury resulting from a direct blow to the anterior thigh, injuring the bony tissue beneath the quadriceps muscle. In the last five years, however, it describes muscles other than the quadriceps. One source, Dr. Max M. Novich, describes charley horse, as "the result of a direct blow to the anterior thigh." Dr. J. V. Cerney describes it as "that involuntary cramping of muscles accompanied by sharp pain and temporary paralysis of that body part." Although there is considerable disagreement as to the mechanics of injury, there is less disagreement, however, as to the approach of treatment.

Signs and Symptoms

1. Pain upon movement
2. Pain during muscle contraction
3. Muscle spasm
4. Tenderness
5. Hemorrhage felt as hard mass
6. Swelling
7. Indications of myositis ossificans formation

Treatment

1. Immediate cold-pack applications.
2. Ethyl chloride applications (spray technique); see method described in previous chapter.

3. After 48 hours, apply whirlpool at 104° F. (Do not aim the turbines to injured area.)

4. Medco-Sonlator application to tolerance.

5. Active assistive R.O.M. proceeded by active and resistive R.O.M.

6. Check for posture and balance.

7. Apply flexible adhesive tape.

Special Notes

1. Do not mistake charley horse for myositis.
2. Do not massage a charley horse.
3. Do not use ICE directly to skin—use cold-pack application.
4. Do not use strapping to immobilize the part—use flexible casting as indicated above, and keep athlete active. Physical therapy should be the same as the procedure used in a contused muscle.

Ruptured Leg Muscle

A ruptured leg muscle is the result of a sudden movement that causes the tearing of few or many muscle fibers after subjected to strain beyond their ability to accommodate.

Etiology

1. Untrained athletes
2. Improper warmup
3. Inadequate calisthenics
4. Violent movements
5. Faulty shoes

Signs and Symptoms

1. Moderate to severe pain of leg.
2. Burning sensation.
3. "Feels like hit with an iron bar."
4. Pain during movement of the foot.
5. Pain on pressure of injured area.

6. Discoloration.
7. "Something went snap."
8. Bulging of the involved muscle.
9. Disability.

Considering all the above signs and symptoms, ascertain the ruptured muscle before you begin treatment.

Immediate treatment

1. Cold applications.
2. Compression ace bandage.
3. Flexible adhesive cast—plaster casting is dependent on the degree of rupture.
4. Non-weight bearing is indicated—have athlete use crutches for the first few days.
5. After 2 or 3 days, begin physical therapy with modalities and mild exercise.
6. Progressive resistive exercise should begin after full excursion of movement has been attained.
7. Mild stretching exercise—to increase the flexibility of the muscle.
8. Flexible casting during mild practice field sessions.

Special Notations

1. The extent of the disability varies between 4 and 8 weeks, depending on the degree and the number of ruptured muscle fibers.
2. Muscle rupture will be complete after 12-48 hours.
3. The leg will be paralyzed when the muscle has been totally ruptured and the tendons torn from their attachments.
4. Distal rupturing bulges on the upper end; proximal rupturing bulges at the lower end (Figure 53).
5. When total rupture occurs it is best treated by surgical repair or plaster-cast immobilization. When the cast is removed, physical-therapy techniques under the orthopedic surgeon's direction, should follow.

In general, when treating muscles, you must remember that atrophy (weakness) from disuse occurs very rapidly. Therefore, the injured muscle should never be placed in complete rest. Mild exercises and stimulation, initially followed by progressive resistive exercises, should continue until the termination of treatment. Exercises encourage local circulation, impede the formation of adhesions, and reduce the chances of deformity.

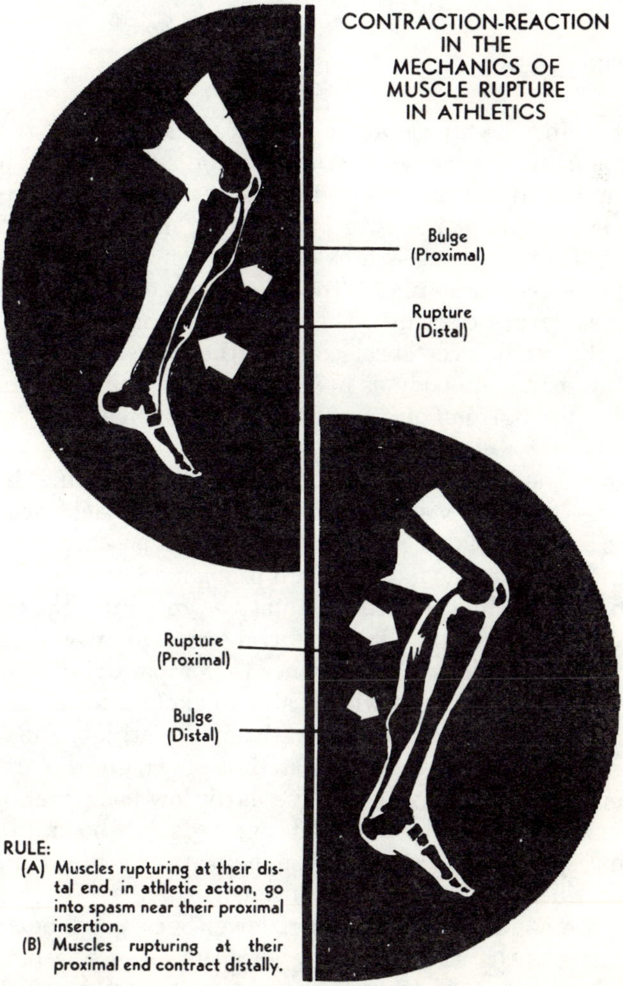

Figure 53. Muscle rupture and its contraction mechanics.

13. Low-Back and Trunk Injuries and Care

General Discussion

The skeleton and the musculature of the back are largely responsible for the support of the trunk, providing stabilization of the upper extremities and head, as well as providing a cushion for the stresses and strains experienced by the lower back during movement of the lower extremities. The enormous strains resulting from the multidirectional movement of soccer accounts for the prevalence of low-back pain. The lumbar musculature consequently becomes enormously important in protecting the lumbar vertebrae column (the lowest five movable vertebrae), stabilizing the body as a whole and providing flexibility and contractility for harmoniously coordinated movement of both lower extremities.

In view of the importance of the lower-back musclature, it becomes quite obvious that injury and crippling of the lower back incapacitates the body as a whole, making mobility and correct posture very difficult and/or painful. One of the most difficult problems related to lower-back injuries in soccer athletes is the evaluative procedure: the difficulties in establishing the correct diagnosis and, consequently, establishing the correct therapeutic procedure. Once the proper diagnosis has been made, the physical therapist will be able to explain to the athlete the degree of his injury and/or procedures that the athlete should follow for maximum results in the shortest time. It should be emphasized that it would be detrimental to have early low-back manipulations and/or heat applications by so-called "specialists" who call these manipulations "spinal adjustments." The majority of athletic injuries occur primarily because of poorly conditioned athletes.

There are a number of causes of lower-back pain, but the most common cause is the strain and pressure placed on the lumbosacral junctions (Figure 54). The lower back is used mostly as a lever, especially in lifting or lowering a weight. The forces acting on the lum-

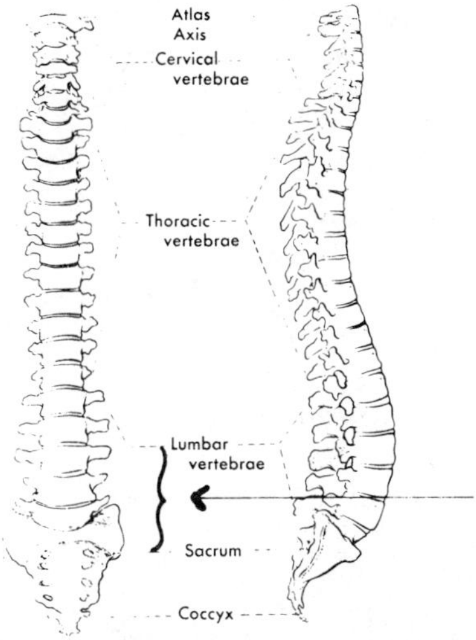

Figure 54. Vertebral Column: Anterior and lateral views as well as Lumbo-Sacral Junction.

bosacral junction may become very great. The estimate is more than two hundred pounds of pressure may be exerted on the lumbosacral disk (that is the cushion between the vertebrae) of an average-sized man making only ordinary movements. The same man, lifting a weight of fifty pounds by straightening his back, can have a pressure of five hundred pounds occur at the lumbosacral junction. It is for this reason, as well as the direct blows received and/or jumping and falling during action on the soccer field, that lower-back pain is relatively common. All types of back pain are caused by some type of irritation, usually affecting the sensory nerve endings. The area of pain may indicate injury to that particular area or refer to an injury from a site nearby. This discrepancy makes if difficult, at times, to identify the exact area of the injury. However, since back problems in soccer athletes are a common injury, every effort must be made to obtain an accurate diagnosis, based on the athlete's own report and the observable signs. Among the things to be considered when recording the athlete's report are:

1. Location of injury
2. Previous history of a similar injury
3. Back pain after strenuous exercise
4. Any chills or hot flashes
5. Back pain after a meal
6. Pain when relaxed

7. Constant pain
8. Type of pain—dull ache or sharp
9. Pain eased by position, heat, cold, pressure, etc.

Signs and Symptoms

1. Redness.
2. Bruises.
3. Swelling.
4. Abnormal bony prominences.
5. Abnormal tissure masses.
6. Abnormal curvature of vertebrae column: a. lordosis, b. scoliosis, c. kyphosis.
7. Foot or arch trouble.
8. Hardened or swollen glands in back of neck.
9. Painful areas along spine during palpation, tapping, or application of pressure.
10. Muscle tightness or distortions.

Keeping the safety and well-being of the player in mind, a course of action must be taken in consultation with the team physician and the team physiotherapist. If this is not done, and the player continues to work out, repeated injuries are likely to occur. Even after a mandatory period of rest between 12 and 24 hours, the injury must be treated with the proper application of physical-therapy modalities followed by exercise, or the injury will require a prolonged rehabilitation.

Sprains

Sprains of the lower back result from overstretching or tearing of the ligaments and muscles in the back. It is important to record the history of the injury and to inspect the injured area. Upon inspection, swelling may not be present, but during palpation, the exact area of pain may be found. There will definitely be a distinction between a sprain of the lumbosacral region and a sacroiliac sprain, although the symptoms may appear to be the same. Symptoms of sacroiliac and lumbosacral sprains are:

1. Muscle spasm of lumbar muscles
2. Decrease of lumbosacral flexibility
3. Decrease and limitation of straight leg raising
4. Local tenderness (higher in the lumbosacral)

5. Tenderness in buttocks, thigh, and leg (sacroiliac)

In reviewing the above symptoms, we see considerable similarity except the fourth and fifth symptoms differ in local tenderness. In the lumbosacral sprain, the pain and tenderness will be found much higher than the sacroiliac joint where the pain will be directly over the joint. The lumbosacral joint is located between movable and immovable portions of the spine and becomes more prone to injury, especially during violent flexion and hyperextension of the spine. The sacroiliac joint, protected by strong ligaments is minimally movable (five degrees the most) and may be injured only by direct blows applied to the joint or by violent rotary movements. The most common symptom that most players experience is localized pain, although pain may be generalized throughout the entire lower back. When the pain becomes exaggerated with movement of the lower extremities (both legs), it will be relieved in most instances by rest. In this case, a firm mattress is indicated. A ¾-inch plywood board under any mattress will be sufficient to provide enough firmness. Muscle spasm usually occurs locally as well as on one or both lower extremities. Usually a spasm will occur on the hamstring group resulting in difficulty flexing the hip with the knee straight. The degree of knee flexion at times determines the severity of the injury: the greater the limitation of hip flexion while the knee is straight, the more serious the injury. (Figure 55)

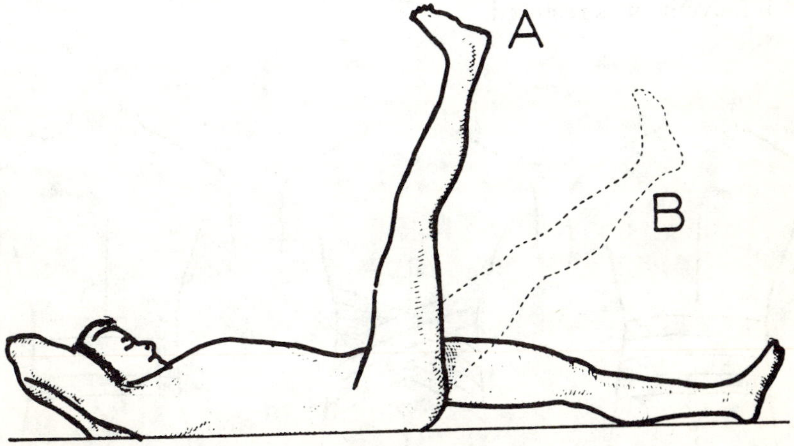

Figure 55. Straight-leg-raising test for sciatic involvement. a. Normal hip flexion b. limited hip flexion indicating sciatic irritation.

Mild Sprain

In mild sprains, the player is able to walk, at times, with a slight limp. Pain will be present during lateral (sideward) or rotary (turning the trunk) movements. Ice applications and/or ethyl chloride spray are indicated immediately after the injury. Strapping (Figure 56) will be of considerable value. Medcosonlator application has been very successful with trigger points and painful muscles spasms of the low back. The application of hydrocollator hot packs after twenty four hours is definitely indicated. Massage should follow the heat application in an attempt to eliminate the tightness of the back muscles and thus promote movement. Therapeutic exercise will follow in the form of William's flexion low-back rationale. This exercise will assist the stretching of the muscles of the lumbar area and the strengthening of the abdominal wall. It will also restore the flexibility of the lumbosacral spine. If the pain lessens during the heat application and increases after the therapeutic exercise, the application of transcutaneous electrical nerve stimulation (T.E.N.S.) is strongly suggested. This new method of treating pain through modified electrical currents has been, in my experience, a very successful method, and I do recommend it strongly.

Thus, to summarize, the treatment of mild sprain should be as follows:

1. Ice pack and/or ethyl chloride spray immediately after injury and for the first 12 hours.

2. Strapping of lumbosacral areas as illustrated, to be continued until movement is restored.

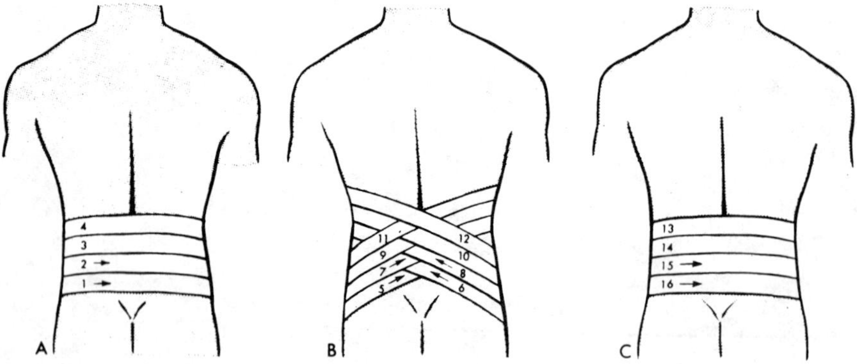

Figure 56. Strapping of low back after mild sprain.

3. Hydrocollator hot packs applications (20 minutes).
4. Massage in the form of petrissage (kneading).
5. Medcosonlator with trigger points.
6. William's Flexion Low Back Exercises (Figures 57, 58, 59, 60, 61a, b, c, d).

The above physical therapy program is to continue twice daily if possible. Approximate time of complete restoration will be between 5 and 7 days.

Moderate Sprain

In moderate sprains, the pain is constant, and the athlete feels uncomfortable most of the time. The rest period is much longer than in a mild sprain. Mild stretching exercises should not be attempted until the pain subsides. A plywood board between the mattress and the springs is helpful. A soft mattress will cause tightening of the back muscles, resulting in considerable pain. Spinal traction for modified home use with water bag and pulleys at the foot of the bed has been used with some success in reducing the muscle spasm. Similar success

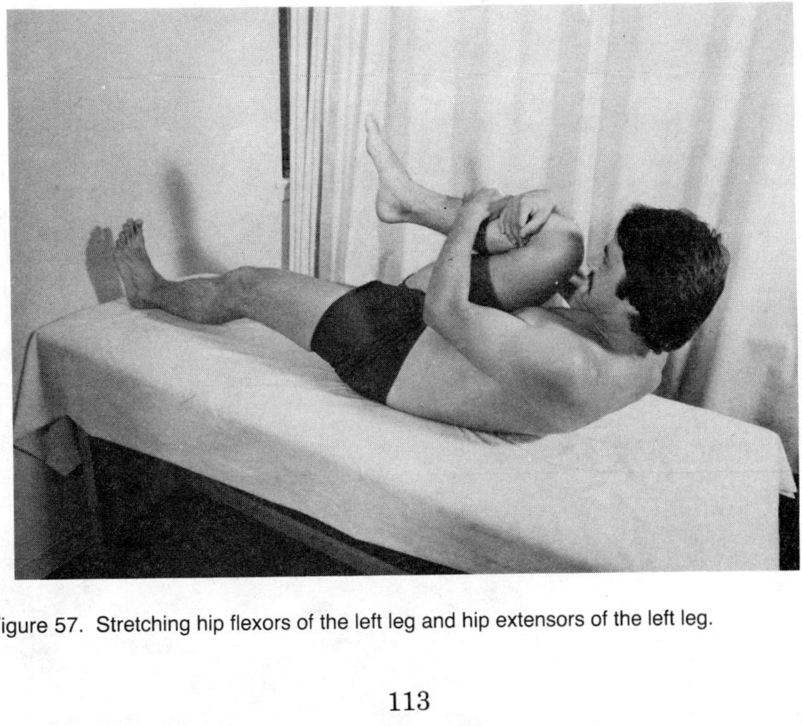

Figure 57. Stretching hip flexors of the left leg and hip extensors of the left leg.

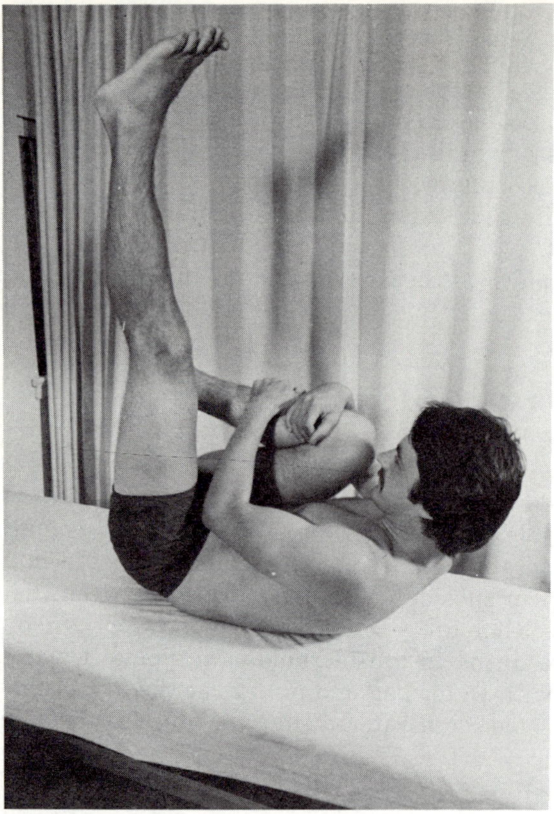

Figure 58. Stretching right hip extensors and left hamstrings.

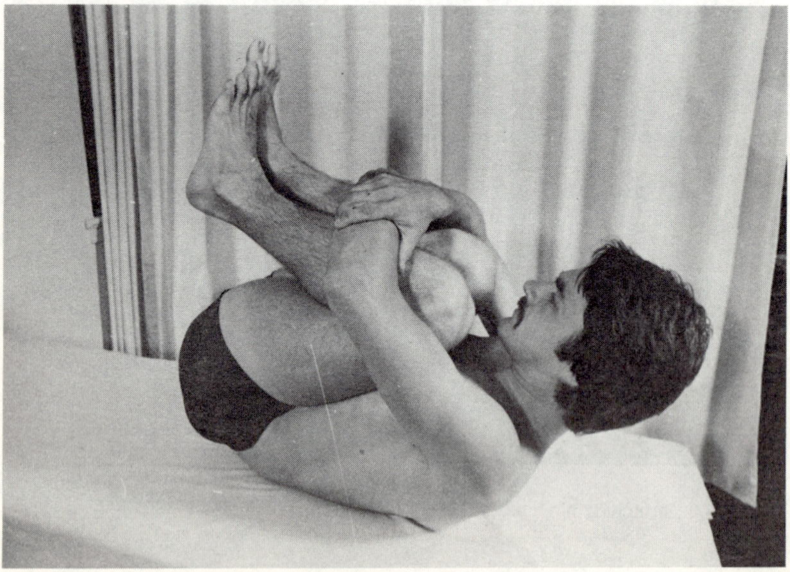

Figure 59. Stretching lumbosacral spine.

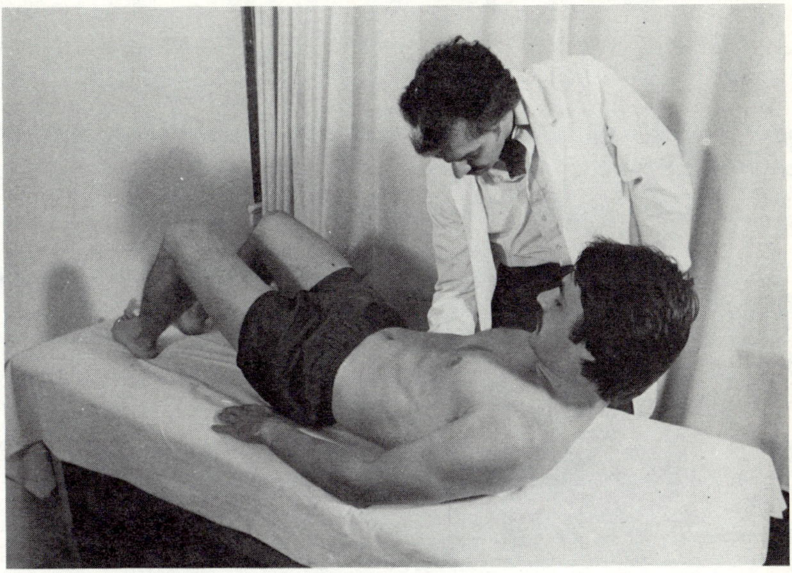

Figure 60. Tightening buttocks and abdominals simultaneously.

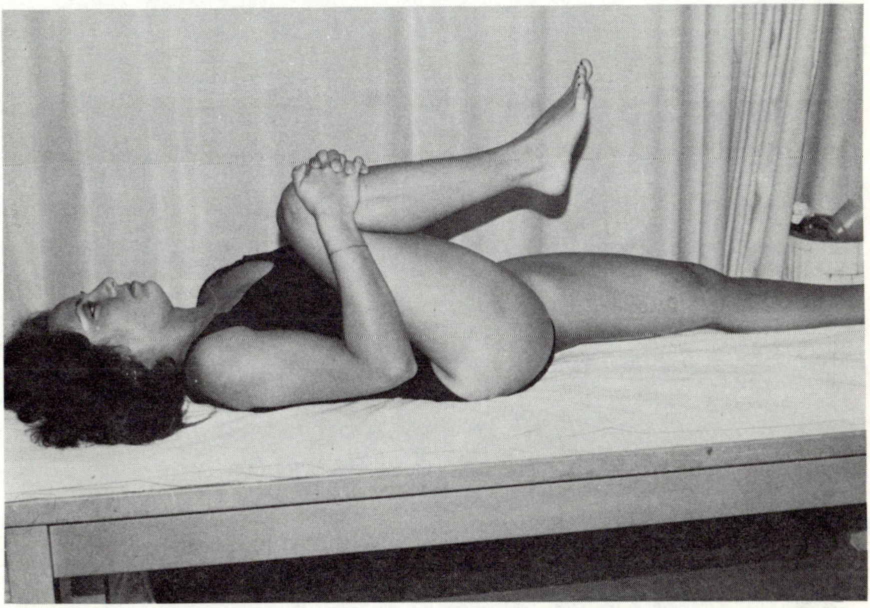

Figure 61a–d. Same as figures 57–60 with slight deviations in view of greater flexibility among female athletes.

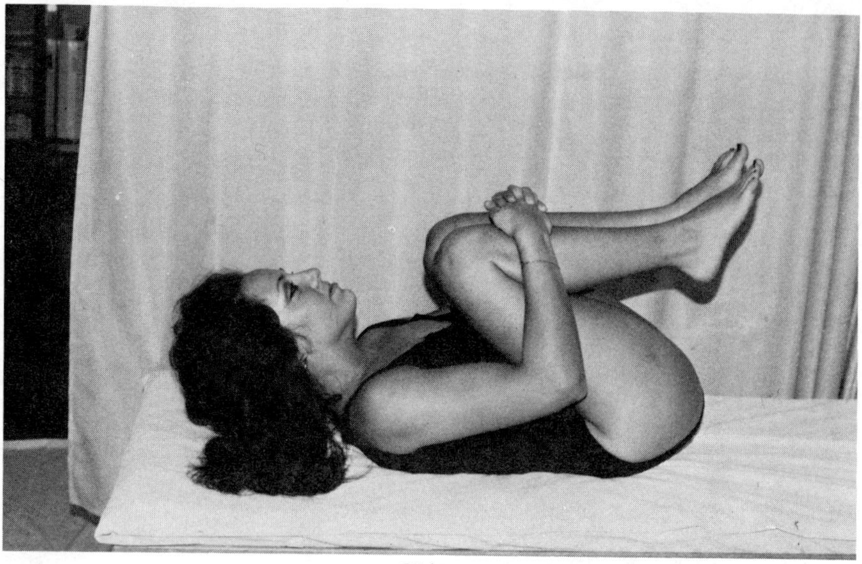

61 b

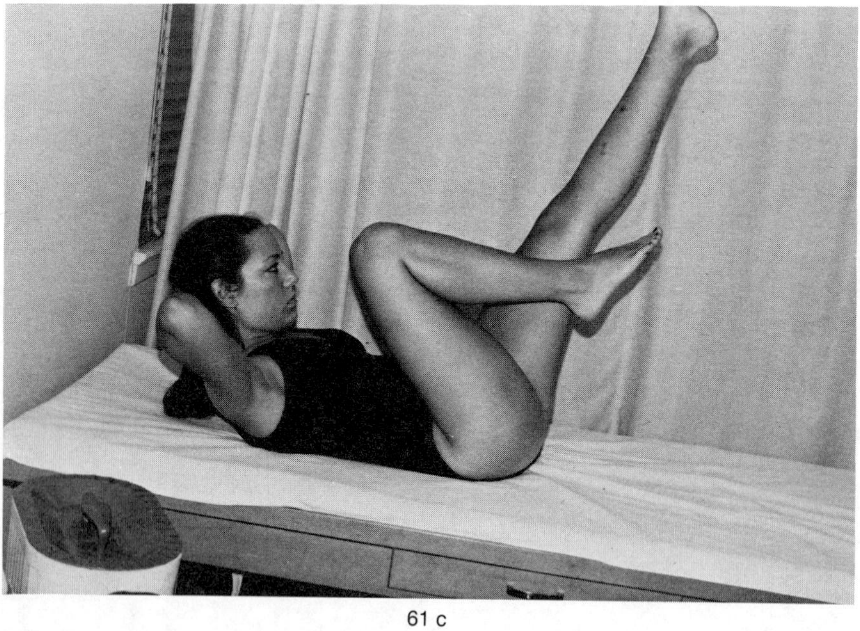

61 c

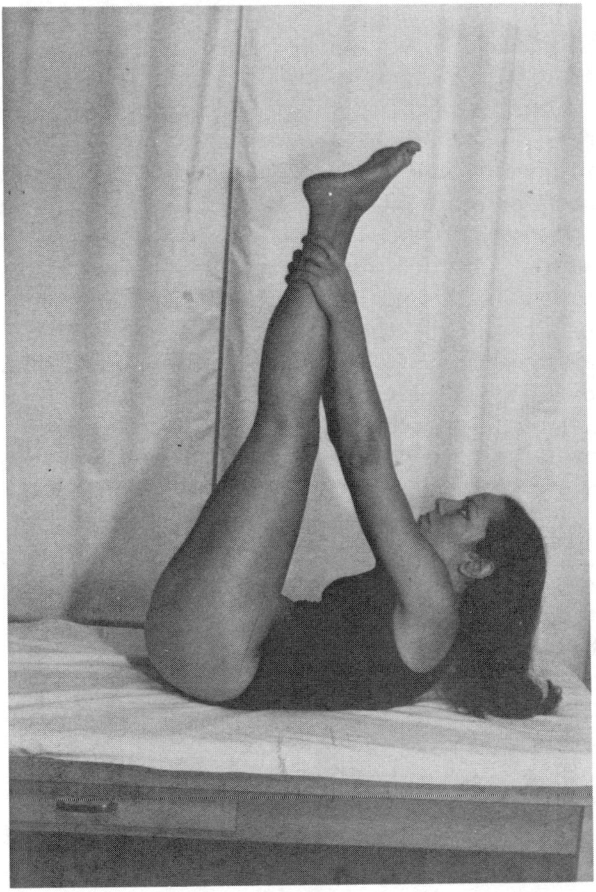

61 d

is achieved by placing a firm pillow under the knees. The pillow, however, should be removed after the initial stage; otherwise, muscle tightness will develop in the hamstring area, which eventually will increase the muscle spasm of the back once the athlete is up on his feet. The immediate treatment will be the same as in mild sprains. X-rays are indicated in order to rule out the possibility of bone involvement. When the symptoms subside, the treatment is the same as in mild sprains.

Severe Sprains

In severe sprains, considerable pain and discomfort are present.

The athlete will be in a state of agony and will not be able to find a comfortable position. There will be radiating pain to one or both legs. This radiating pain is thought to be due to an irritation of the nerve roots of the lumbosacral plexus or to a protrusion of a ruptured intervertebrae disk (cushion between vertebrae bodies) (Figures 62a, b). This radiating pain usually follows the distribution of the sciatic nerve, causing irritation of the leg as well as, at times, numbness or hyperesthesia (hypersensitivity to touch).

During first aid, the athlete should be removed from the field by competent professionals and taken to the emergency care at the nearest hospital for x-rays. Once the x-rays have ruled out the possibility of fracture, and the physician has prescribed the proper analgesics, bed rest is indicated, and pelvic traction must be considered. The team physician should then advise the physical therapist the course of action after the initial rest stage, which might last between 24 and 48 hours. The course of treatment to follow afterward should be the same as in moderate sprains.

Special Note: Back injuries mostly occur in poorly conditioned athletes who maintain their "anatomic corset," namely, the abdominal musculature and the back and hip extensors, in poor shape.

Contusions

The muscles of the back, especially the upper gluteals (buttocks),

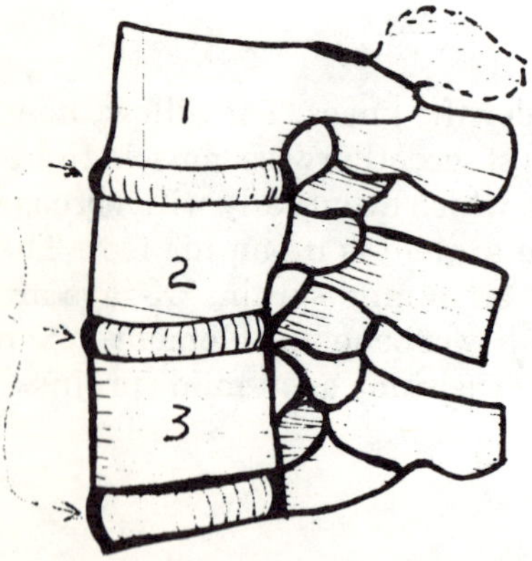

Figure 62a. Normal intervertebral cushion.

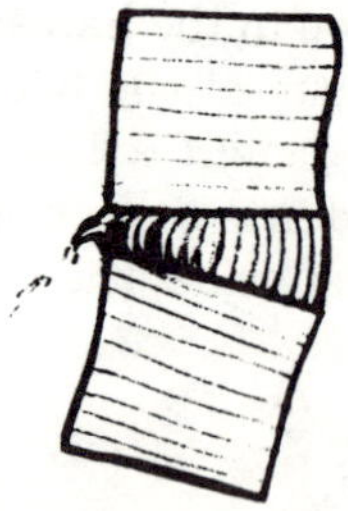

Figure 62b. Ruptured disk (cushion).

are subject to bruising resulting from direct blows from kicks, chops with an elbow, or slamming against a goal post. The contusion of the gluteals can be a very disabling condition, keeping the athlete out of competition for a considerable time. The injury will involve considerable pain and discomfort during movement but will be free of pain during rest. In a severe contusion, the athlete has difficulty in walking or standing. A thorough examination to eliminate the possibility of bone involvement is necessary. Once the examination and/or the x-ray have ruled out any possibility of bone involvement, the immediate care of the injury should consist of the following:

1. Ice-pack application.
2. Strapping for compression to tolerance.
3. Heat applications, after hemorrhage has been controlled—usually after 5 days.
4. Medcosonlator to tolerance.
5. Kneading massage to buttocks.
6. Therapeutic exercise to eliminate tightness and promote strength to abdominals and hip extensors.

The athlete should not resume any activity before full range of motion has been attained. The length of disability varies between 2 days and 2 weeks.

Special Note: In view of the large area of muscle bulk and the vast blood supply to this area, contusion to this muscle may be a problem. A compression bandage and application of ice cannot be applied very satisfactorily. The application of an elastic strapping or other means of compression have not been too successful in view of the location of the buttocks. Therefore, bed rest, ice-pack application, and mild therapeutic exercise starting the third day should be the treatment of choice, especially for a severe gluteal contusion.

Contusions of the kidneys should always be considered when treating back injuries. After carefully listening to the athlete and locating the injury, a kidney contusion should not be eliminated until the athlete's urine has been examined by the team's physician. The kidneys are located on the posterior (back) region, extending on either side of the lowest thoracic and first three lumbar vertebrae (Figure 63). Any direct blow to this region should always be checked for possible injury to the kidneys.

Lumbago

Lumbago is the term used for any pain and discomfort to the

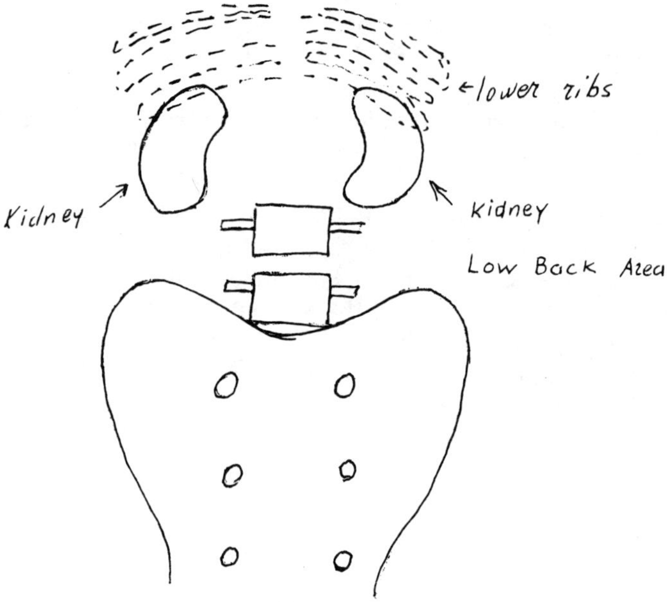

Figure 63. Demonstrates location of kidneys.

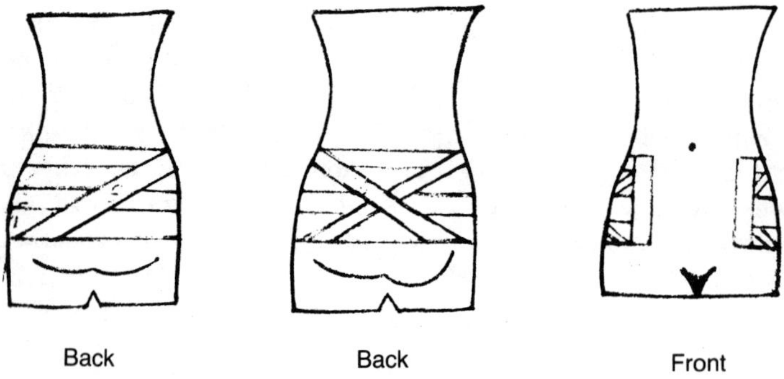

Figure 64. Strapping of low back.

lumbar muscles of the back. Other common terms used to describe this condition are "fibrositis," "myositis," or "sacroiliac disease." In athletic injuries, when this term is used, it refers usually to a fibrositic condition of the muscles of the low back.

Signs and Symptoms

1. Dull aching pain across low back.
2. Inability to bend or stoop.
3. Inability to turn due to pain.
4. Pain during movements of lower extremities.

Treatment

1. Ice packs during initial stage.
2. Medcosonlator with trigger points to tolerance.
3. Ethyl chloride spray to trigger points.
4. Medcollator application with pulsating currents.
5. Moist heat after third day.
6. Kneading massage.
7. Therapeutic exercises, including stretching and strengthening to the back muscles and abdominals, respectively.
8. Strapping of the lower back.

Strapping in lower-back injuries is very important in the initial stages of the injury as well as during practice sessions. Strapping of the lower back is demonstrated in Figure 64. The athlete is standing with his feet apart approximately 16 inches. A pretape material is wrapped around his waist to prevent skin irritations. Use 2-inch-thickness adhesive tape.

Step 1. The first strip on the abdomen above the pelvis, and pull the tape tight across the back below the sacrum to the same position as the start except on the opposite side of the pelvis.

Step 2. Repeat the above step, overlapping halfway from the beginning to the end. The extent of the injury will determine the number of strips to be used horizontally.

Step 3. Diagonal strips will be used as reinforcements. Pull a diagonal strip from the lower front and proceed diagonally to the upper position of the opposite side.

Step 4. Reverse the procedure and start from the opposite side.

Step 5. Two or more diagonal strips can be used, overlapping at least halfway. In most cases, two diagonal strips are sufficient.

Step 6. Apply anchor strips to the opposite ends to prevent any slipping or rolling of the tape.

"Low Back"

Low-back injuries can be very disabling and may cause physical and emotional manifestations. At times, the athlete with such manifestations may be accused of being lazy, unmotivated, or even hypochondriacal. Under no circumstances should anyone who is involved with such an athlete underestimate, or become indifferent to, the athlete's so called "faulty" emotions. It is the fault of those who have become indifferent to such injuries and do not bother to know more about them rather than the athlete's physical and emotional manifestations.

14. Shoulder Injuries and Care

General Discussion

The shoulder is a complicated structure made of numerous bones, joints, ligaments, and muscles. It is a highly movable structure; in fact, it is the most mobile joint in the body. Although the shoulder joint is formed by the articular surfaces of only two bones, glenohumeral joint, comprised of the glenoid cavity and the head of the humerus, its movement, however, is dependent on the synchronous normal movement of three other joints: the acromioclavicular, the sternoclavicular, and the scapulochest wall joints (Figures 65a, b). The last joint is not a synovial joint, but for functional purposes it acts as one, especially when the glenohumeral joint is impaired. The bony components of the shoulder include the clavicle, the head of the humerus, the scapula, the sternum, and the portion of the posterior thorax where the scapula moves.

The shoulder joint is a ball and socket joint and allows free move-

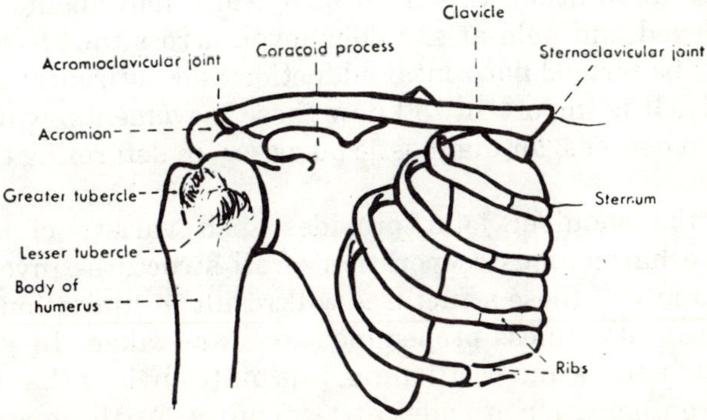

Figure 65a. Shoulder joint, anterior view.

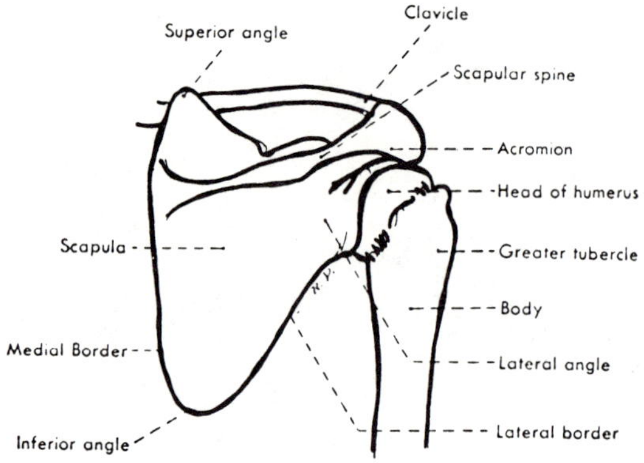

Figure 65b. Skeletal anatomy of the shoulder joint (posterior view).

ments such as abduction, adduction, flexion, extension, rotation, and the combined movements of circumduction. These movements for practical purposes will be defined in terms of the body as a whole rather than in relationship to the scapula. Thus, flexion of the shoulder is a forward movement of the arm. Extension is the reverse movement, the return from flexion and backward movement of the arm. Abduction is the raising of the arm laterally away from the body; adduction, the return from abduction or bringing the arm to the side. Circumduction is a combination of all of the above movements, resulting in describing a circle with the arm. Internal rotation or medial rotation is the movement of the arm about its long axis with the elbow held in flexion and palm facing down at shoulder level. A downward and backward movement along the humeral axis will be termed medial rotation, while the opposite—upward and backward—along the humeral axis will be termed lateral rotation. Simultaneously, any movement, while the elbow is flexed and held at shoulder level, across the chest or away from it will be termed horizontal adduction and horizontal abduction, respectively. It is important to know these movements, which can be expressed in degrees, for diagnostic purposes, in determing the degree of injury.

Since the shoulder joint provides such variety of movement through the harmonious cooperation of all structures involved, any violation to any of these structures will result in limitation and consequent disability unless proper measures are taken. In view of its anatomic structures and positioning, it is quite obvious that the shoulder's bony configuration provides little stability. Furthermore, the capsular ligaments permitting such wide range of movement provide hardly any opposition to forces acting on the shoulder joint. Consequently, it is the muscles and tendons of the shoulder joint that play an essential role not only in providing mobility but stability as well. Therefore, in preventing shoulder injuries, proper care must begin with conditioning the surrounding muscles of the shoulder rather than the applications of protective measures.

Signs and Symptoms

1. Localized and occasionally generalized pain depending on the injured area
2. Generalized tenderness
3. Limitation in range of motion
4. Athlete's favoring an arm
5. Swelling
6. Apprehension

Functional Tests

1. Look at injured shoulder and observe any abnormalities when compared to opposite shoulder.
   a. Check all sides and compare contours.
   b. Any change in contour may point out fracture, dislocation or sublaxations.
   c. Any obvious deformity should suggest the immediate attention of team's physician.
2. Palpate the area of injury gently. The bones of the shoulder are easily palpable.
   a. Ask athlete to move his shoulder gently.
   b. Don't attempt any rough movement.
   c. Check actively the movements of neighboring joints such as elbow, wrist, and hand grasp.
   d. Ask athlete to form a fist or to bend elbow.
3. When any serious injury is ruled out, ask athlete to perform actively all the movements permitted by the shoulder, the ones discussed earlier in this chapter.
4. Limitation in any of the movements would most probably pinpoint the injured muscle. The following procedure should be performed when testing for muscle injury.
   a. Raise arm sideways—this is a test for shoulder abduction primarily performed by the middle deltoid.

b. Lower arm from horizontal position—when some resistance is applied, it is a test for latissimus dorsi and teres major and possibly posterior deltoid.

c. Hyperextend the arm backward. This is a test for posterior deltoid and teres minor and major.

d. Swing the arm forward or shoulder flexion. This tests anterior deltoid and the coracobrachialis, supported by the pectoralis major and biceps.

e. Rotate the arm at shoulder level with elbow bent; the forearm is moved downward for medial rotation. This tests the subscapularis, pectoralis major, and latissimus dorsi.

f. Rotate arm at shoulder level as above with forearm moving upward as in external rotation. This tests infraspinatus and teres minor.

Dislocation

Dislocation of the shoulder joint may be defined as the total displacement of one articular surface from another. Partial dislocation will be the result of incomplete displacement, also known as subluxation. Although shoulder injuries are not too common in soccer, dislocations, however, are the most common of shoulder injuries. The reason for this is the construction of the joint, as discussed earlier, as well as the degree of hypermobility. Physical therapy is very important and should start immediately to avoid any complications resulting from immobilization. Once the nature of dislocation has been established regarding anterior or posterior displacement, the faster the reduction of pain and the sooner the athlete will feel comfortable.

Until the physician reduces the dislocation, the injured athlete's arm should be placed in a sling. There are two very popular methods of reducing a dislocation: (1) the Kocher's method, used by many trainers, and (2) the foot in axilla method, used by many physicians. I would, however, suggest neither of the above. I would recommend that the athlete be sent to emergency care for x-rays to rule out the possibility of any other bone pathology, and while there, the shoulder should be reduced by a *physician* (orthopedic surgeon).

After reduction, a flexible cast should be applied as demonstrated in Figure 67. The principle of this taping is to pull the shoulder up with the tape and not by the athlete's own muscle strength. This method of strapping can be modified in a more severe dislocation by extending the tape to the opposite side as demonstrated in Figure 68.

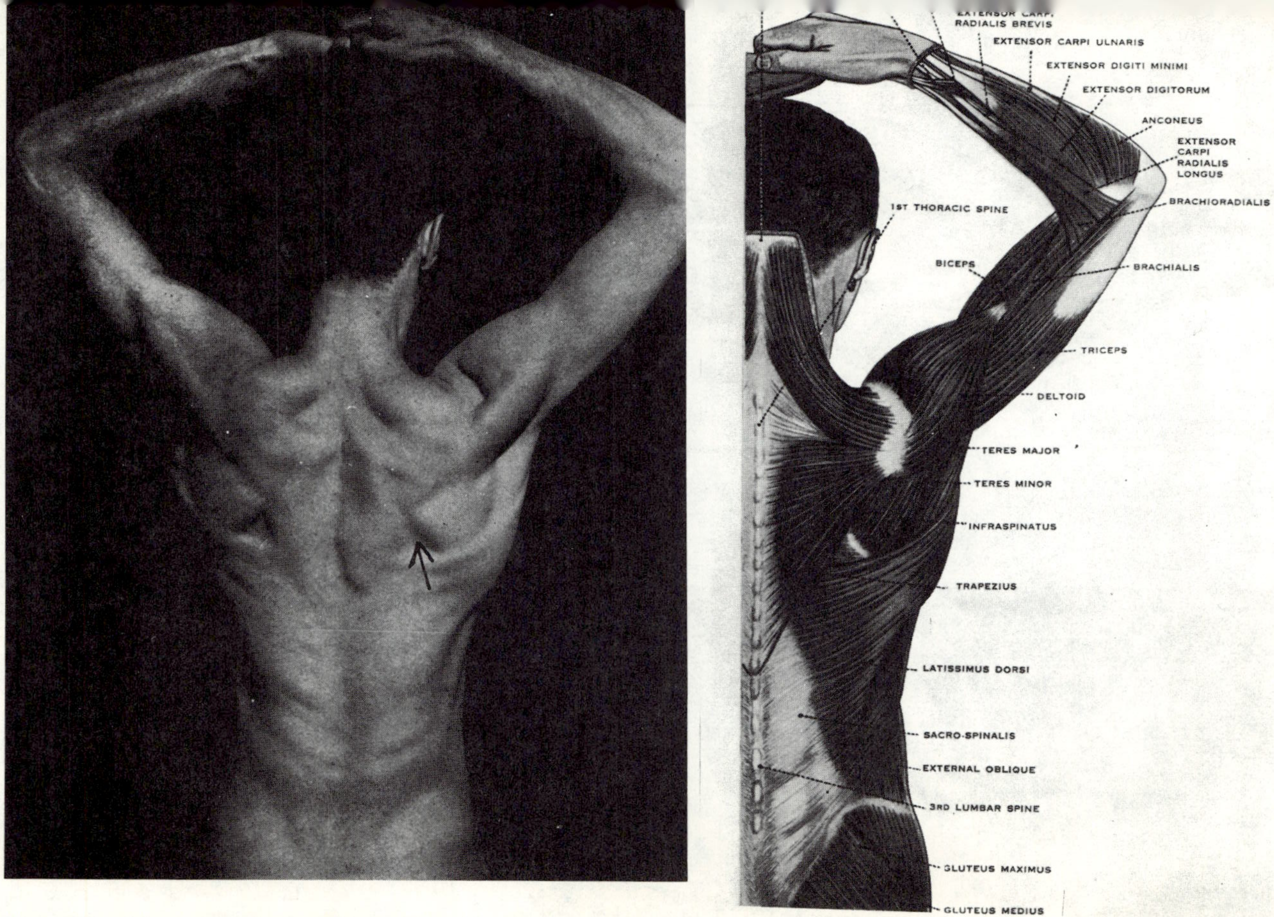

Figure 66a. Muscles on the shoulder and scapula.

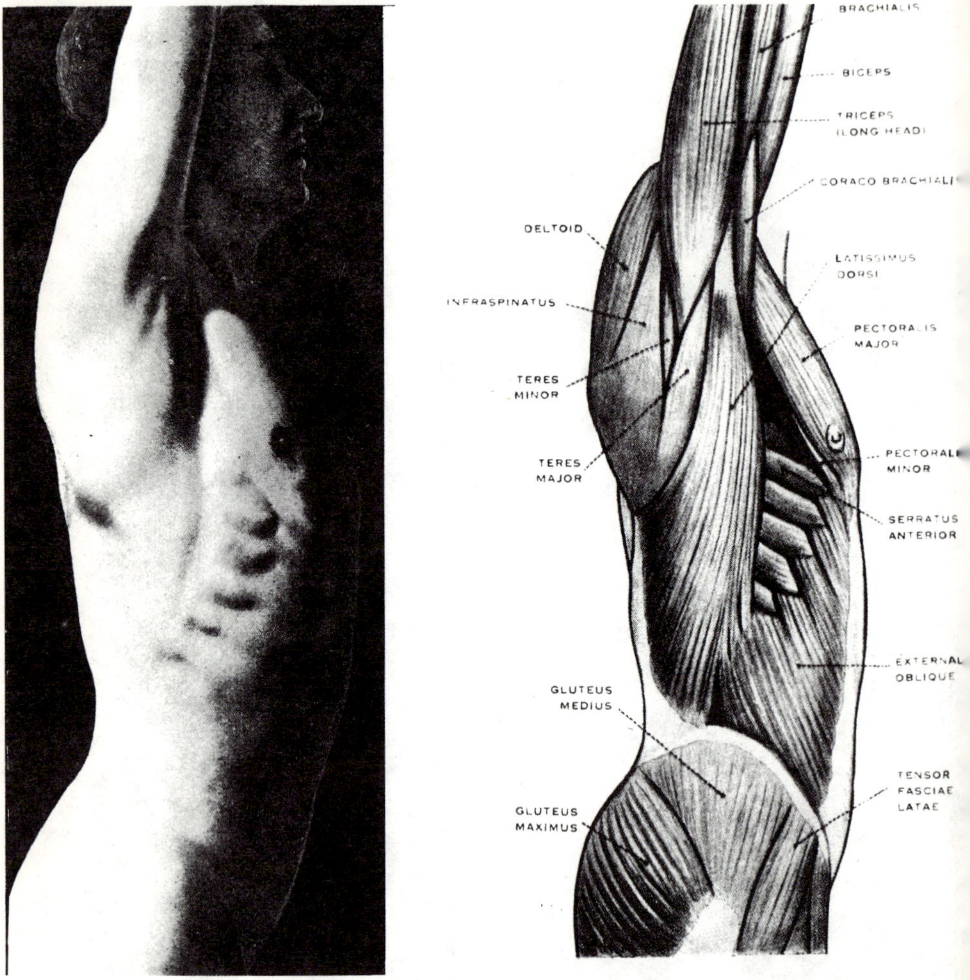

Figure 66b. Anterior and lateral muscles of the shoulder joint.

The terminology, mild, moderate, and severe dislocation pertains to the degree of displacement of the head of the humerus anteriorly, posteriorly, downward, or upward. The anterior dislocation occurs more frequently and is not as severe as the posterior dislocation. A partial displacement of the head of the humerus will be termed a mild dislocation or subluxation. Any form of moderate or severe dislocation results in the tear of the capsule, the stretching of the ligaments and muscles, and, in some cases, the tearing of the muscles. The history

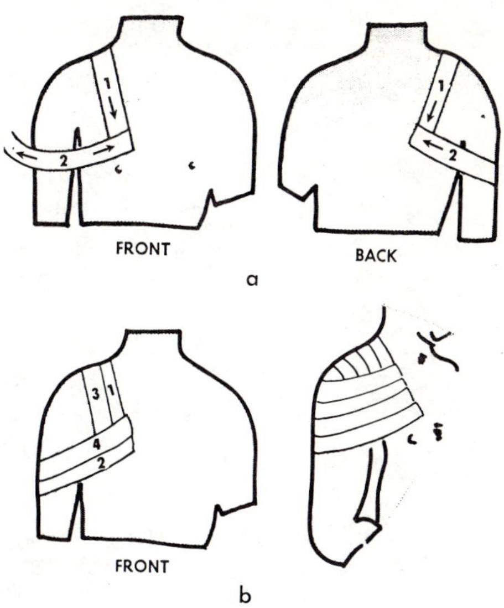

Figure 67. Flexible cast as demonstrated after the shoulder has been reduced.

given by the athlete, the functional tests as well as the signs and symptoms, will help in establishing the degree of injury.

Initial Treatment

1. X-rays to cancel out any possibility of fracture.
2. Reduction of the displacement.
3. Flexible cast as illustrated.
4. Ice application for the first 24–48 hours.
5. Mild active isometric exercises of the elbow, forearm, wrist, and hand grasp.
6. Active assistive R.O.M. after the fifth day; stop if pain and discomfort persist.

Follow-up Treatment

1. Moist heat.
2. Gentle active assistive R.O.M.
3. Transcutaneus nerve stimulation.

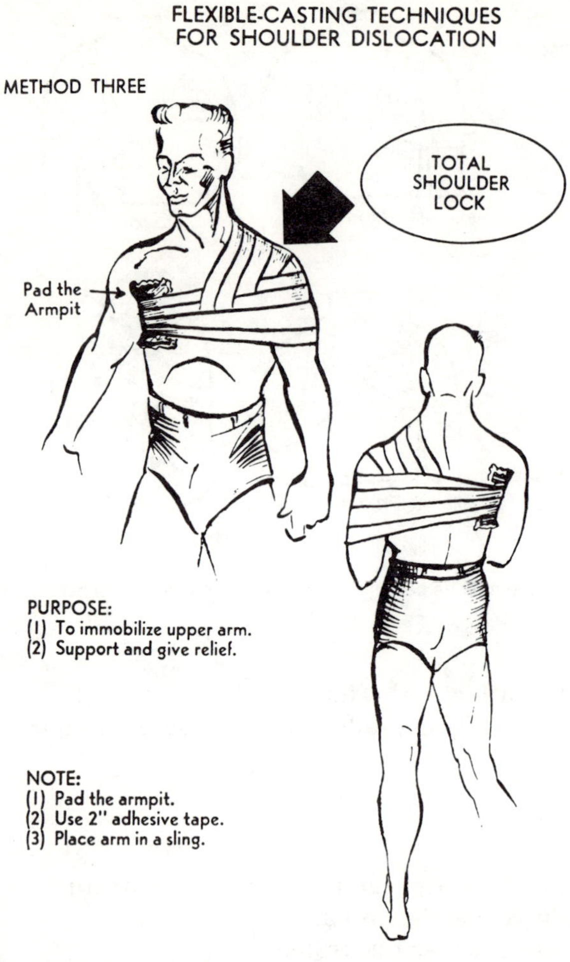

Figure 68. Extensive flexible casting after severe dislocation.

4. Pendulum exercises.
5. Progressive resistive exercises to elbow flexion and extension.

Special Note: For the first 3–5 weeks, you must avoid full abduction and rotation of the shoulder. Even after 6 weeks' time, when full rehabilitation is expected, the athlete should continue to protect the shoulder during field activity with a special shoulder harness, available at surgical supplies stores.

The muscles of the shoulder are large, covering the upper part of the body from all directions: anteriorly, posteriorly and laterally. Anteriorly, the most prominent muscles are the pectorals, whose prime movement has been described earlier in this chapter. Other muscles anteriorly and laterally are: pectoralis minor, anterior deltoid, trapezius (upper fibers), sternocleidomastoideus and serratus anterior. Posteriorly, the most prominent muscles are the trapezii, whose main function is to adduct the scapula (middle fibers), elevate the shoulder (upper fibers) and depress the scapula (lower fibers). Other muscles of the posterior surface that act on the shoulder are: posterior deltoid, posterior fibers of serratus, teres major, latissimus dorsi, teres minor, infraspinatus, supraspinatus, and rhomboideus. (Figures 66a, b) The function of the above muscles has been described earlier in this chapter. In view of the large size of these muscles and their dependency on each other in producing a movement at the shoulder, any injury to any group of muscles will involve the function of the shoulder and, consequently, the movements produced by the elbow and, to a lesser extent, by the hand. In addition, injury to the muscles, with attachments to the anterior, posterior, and lateral wall of the thorax, will impede such functions as deep inspiration and/or deep expiration of the thoracic cavity. Physical therapy consequently plays a major role in the rehabilitation of the shoulder in the initial stages of first aid as well as the follow-up care.

Initial Stages

1. For the first 24–48 hours, the application of ice packs and a flexible cast is essential.
2. After the 48 hours, applications of heat, which will act as a pain reliever.
3. Isometric exercises to maintain the muscle tone.
4. Mild effleurage to enhance the local metabolism and reduce the local muscle spasm.
5. Active range of motion of the adjacent joints such as elbow, forearm, wrist, and fingers.
6. Breathing exercises to maintain the contractility of the chest muscles, thus enhancing the movements of the thoracic cavity.

Follow-up Care of the Shoulder

During this period, since the pain of the shoulder has been decreased considerably, attention should be directed toward the reestablishment of shoulder movement and the reeducation of muscle strength. To reestablish the joint movement, we use the following modalities: (1) ultrasound for 5–10 minutes, (2) short-wave diathermy for 20 minutes, (3) deep massage in the form of petrissage, and (4) transcutaneous nerve stimulation.

For Muscle reeducation

1. Active assistive R.O.M.
2. Active R.O.M.
3. Active resistive and progressive resistive R.O.M.

Note: The movements must be gently firm but not rough. Progressive resistive exercise should begin after the pain has diminished and the R.O.M. has been actively completed.

4. Pendulum exercises and wheel exercises with resistance are advocated once complete R.O.M. has been established.

Note: The return of the athlete to field practice is a very delicate matter, and the decision depends on the cooperation of the coach, the physician, the physical therapist, and the athlete himself. The latter should make the final decision once all therapeutic interventions have been exhausted.

Contusions

Shoulder contusion is not that common among soccer players. When they do occur, either by direct blows to the shoulder or by falling into a hard surface, they mainly involve the deltoid muscle, which encases the shoulder joint anteriorly, posteriorly, and laterally. A shoulder contusion is that injury that causes laceration and tearing without breaking the continuity of the overlying skin. The most common place of such contusion is at the area of the acromioclavicular joint.

Signs and Symptoms

1. Tight shoulder that "stiffens up."
2. Limitation in R.O.M.
3. Swelling.
4. Local heat.

5. Sensory loss (sensory nerve injury).

Treatment (immediately after injury)

1. Application of ice pack.
2. Flexible casting (all flexible adhesive).
3. Application of sling.

After 48 Hours:

1. Removal of flexible cast.
2. Moist heat application for 20 minutes.
3. Medcollator pulsating current.
4. Active R.O.M. in all directions.
5. Progressive resistive exercises when complete R.O.M. has been attained.

Note: When player returns to field activity, protective strapping should be applied.

Shoulder Strain

Shoulder strain is very common along the deltoid muscle, which encases the shoulder in all directions. It mainly occurs during a sudden movement where the deltoid is stretched beyond its normal limit. Contusions and muscle strains usually occur among goal keepers where unexpected movements and falls on the ground are quite common.

In a mild strain of the shoulder, the initial application of an ice pack and protective strapping for the first 24 hours may be sufficient with no further treatment necessary. Indeed, heat applications and active R.O.M. will definitely induce the healing process. However, the athlete may regain complete movement without the necessity of heat applications. In a moderate to severe strain, however, the applications of a flexible cast, sling, and ice packs are indicated routinely. For flexible casting in a moderate and severe strain of the shoulder see Figure 69.

Frozen Shoulder

A "frozen shoulder" is painfully limited stiffness of the shoulder resulting from any untreated injury of this region but is mainly associated with rupture or strain of the supraspinatus muscle. I have

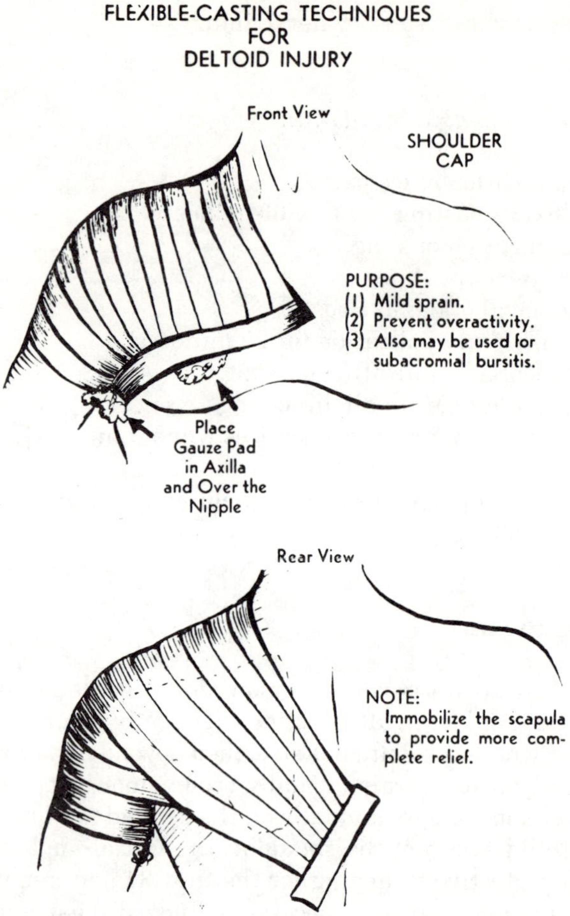

Figure 69. Flexible casting for deltoid and pectoral injury.

simply mentioned this injury only as a warning to the soccer players who might overindulge themselves with prolonging rest of their injured shoulder. I have never yet treated a total "frozen shoulder" in my experience with soccer injuries.

Etiology

1. Prolonged immobilization after a shoulder injury.
2. Injury or bruising to supraspinatus.

Treatment

1. Moist heat; short-wave Diathermy.
2. Deep massage (petrissage).
3. Manipulation progressively.
4. Electrical stimulation.
5. Reciprocal innervation.
6. Ultrasound around the joint.

Ruptured Muscles

Ruptured muscles seldom occur among soccer players with the exception of the goalkeeper. I must repeat the same statement that I have made with previous injuries. "Prevention is better than correction" and, therefore, regular workouts, calisthenics, stretching, and strengthening exercises, as well as practice field sessions will be the best preventive methods, and the chances of injury will be held to a very minimum. When ruptured muscles do occur, the muscles most commonly injured are the following: pectoralis major, pectoralis minor, deltoid, rotator cuff, biceps, serratus anterior, and triceps.

Pectoralis Major

A ruptured pectoralis major is simply a tearing of the muscle either from its origin (the sternum and/or the medial part of the collar bone) or its insertion (the bicipital groove of humerus). (Figure 70b) The best treatment, even for the most ambitious and enthusiastic player, will be complete rest until healing takes place. Should any forceful movements be applied, they will extend the rupture and increase the disability. Complete healing, depending on the degree of tearing, takes between five days and three weeks.

Treatment (First 24 hours)

1. Locate, by palpation, area of injury.
2. Application of ice pack.
3. Bandage over the ice pack with elbow of involved arm flexed and bandaged against side of the body and across the chest.

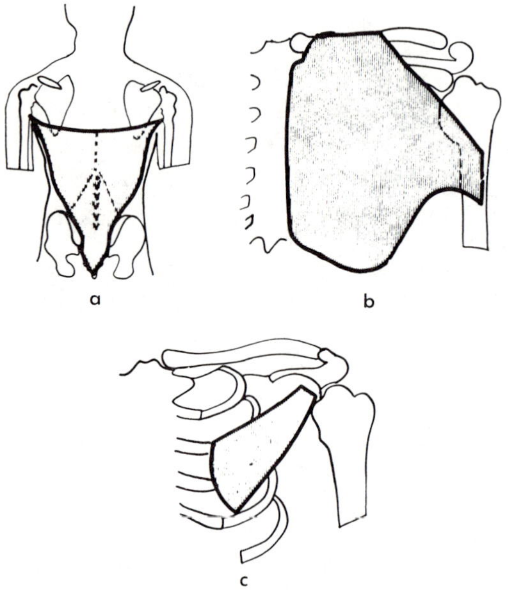

Figure 70a. Long back muscle extending from the shoulder blades downward (Latissimus Dorsi);
Figure 70b. Chest muscle covering most of the rib cage in front (Pectoralis Major);
Figure 70c. Deep muscle, Pectoralis Minor.

Treatment (After 24 hours)

1. Application of heat—preferably moist (hydrocollator hot packs) for 20–30 minutes.
2. Mild massage around the injured area (not over the injury).
3. Slight active-assistive movement using pain as guide.
4. Shoulder strap with sling.
5. Complete rest from workouts involving arm and shoulder.
6. The athlete is permitted to run around the field with the arm and shoulder strapped to his chest.

Note: Passive movements, with the assistance of the athlete's good arm, are permitted very gently to the point of minimum discomfort and not any further. For complete healing, the arm must be strapped and rested on a sling with the elbow flexed throughout the day except during the time of passive gentle exercise.

Pectoralis Minor (Figure 70c)

This muscle is located under the pectoralis major on the front part of the chest. This muscle's origin is from the third, fourth, and fifth rib and inserts into the coracoid process of the scapula. During contraction, this muscle acts as a depressor and lateral rotator of the scapula. A rupture of the pectoralis major may injure the pectoralis minor as well. It occurs very rarely, but when it does, its treatment is similar to that of pectoralis major.

Note: Both the pectoralis major and minor in view of their origin and insertion on the chest cavity are also accessory breathing muscles. Breathing exercises, therefore, are advised after 24 hours as a means of rehabilitating the muscles with gentle inhaling and exhaling with the expansion of the chest.

Rotator Cuff

Rotator cuff pertains to three muscles whose main function is to hold the humerus into the glenoid fossa. These muscles are: the infraspinatus, the teres minor, and the subscapularis. The first two muscles act as external rotators of the shoulder, while the last, the subscapularis, acts as an internal rotator of the shoulder along with the pectoralis major and the latissimus dorsi (Figure 70a). The most common sign during a rupture of any of the rotators is the forced rotation of the arm either inwardly or outwardly according to the ruptured muscle. The athlete will most probably pinpoint the area of the injury.

Treatment (First 24 hours)

1. Flexible strapping.
2. Ice-pack application.
3. Application of sling with flexed elbow.

Treatment (After 24 hours)

1. Application of moist heat, 20–30 minutes.
2. Gentle massage.
3. Gentle movements to the point of mild discomfort.

4. Rest.
5. Strap shoulder at all times except during treatment.
6. After complete healing has taken place and complete R.O.M. is possible, proceed with progressive resistive exercises.
7. Reciprocal innervation techniques are advocated as applied under the supervision of a physical therapist. These techniques have been discussed in an earlier chapter.
8. The athlete should not attend strenuous workouts until complete healing has taken place as when compared with opposite shoulder.

Biceps

Biceps tearing is defined as the loss of the continuity of this muscle as a result of a sudden and excessive pull.

Signs and Symptoms

1. Snapping sound felt in the shoulder.
2. Shoulder pain.
3. Swelling in the biceps.
4. Discoloration.
5. Tenderness.
6. Muscle atrophy.
7. Lack of movement initially.

Treatment (First 24 hours)

1. Cold-pack application.
2. Flexible casting.
3. Sling.
4. Rest.

Treatment (After 24 hours)

1. Moist heat.
2. Pulsating currents (Medcollator).
3. Massage (effleurage).
4. Gentle active-assistive R.O.M.

5. Active R.O.M. when pain subsides.

6. After complete movement free of pain has been attained, start progressive resistive exercise with weights under professional supervision.

Note: An overambitious athlete might attempt unsupervised weightlifting too early and thereby increase the degree of disability and consequently, prolong the recovery period.

Deltoid

This muscle is shaped triangularly, as its name indicates (delta means triangular), and it covers the shoulder in three areas: anteriorly, posteriorly, and laterally. When all its fibers contract, they abduct the arm (raise arm upward from the side). The anterior fibers assist in lifting the arm forward. The posteriors assist in shoulder extension or bringing the arm back from flexion. The middle fibers lift the arm (abduct) sideways. The action of each group of fibers should be known in order to pinpoint the area and extent of injury. The treatment is similar, as in the previous injuries, for the first 24 hours as well as the follow-up. *Strapping* of the shoulder and *rest* should be emphasized. Progressive resistive exercise should be attempted only when complete active R.O.M. free of pain has been attained.

Serratus Anterior

This muscle originates from the outer borders of the upper nine ribs and inserts into the ventral surface of the vertebrae border of the scapula. Its action is to abduct the scapula (bringing it away from the vertebrae border) and to reach forward while arm is at shoulder level. In view of its anatomic position and its attachment to nine ribs, most of the injuries to the serratus are associated with injuries to the ribs. The limitations will affect the abduction of the scapula and the humerus as well as the ability to reach forward (a diagnostic sign). Deep breathing will be painful caused by excessive movement of the thoracic cavity. Treatment will be symptomatic according to the area of injury and the degree of limitation. The therapeutic rationale should be to minimize pain and discomfort, increase the range of motion, and eventually reeducate to its optimum the muscle strength. The last two should begin after the initial treatment of the first 24 hours, which should include: ice applications, strapping, sling, and rest.

Triceps

This muscle is located on the back of the arm just opposite the biceps and has three different heads. The long head originates from the scapula; the lateral head originates from the upper lateral part of the humerus; the medial head originates from the lower posterior part of the humerus. The insertion is at the olecranon process of the ulna. The action of this muscle is to extend the elbow. A rupture of this muscle will obviously prevent the athlete from extending his elbow during the initial stages of his injury. The long head of the triceps will be the only one involved with the functions of the shoulder. The other two heads of the triceps will be mostly involved with the function of the elbow, in the movement of elbow extension. During the first 24 hours, the treatment should be in the form of ice-pack application and strapping of the upper arm. The elbow should *remain straight.* Any flexion of the elbow will stretch the triceps, cause pain and discomfort, and increase the disability. The elbow should be strapped in a very minimal amount of flexion—approximately 10 degrees.

Note: Shoulder exercises will be discussed in greater detail in the final part of this book under the title of "General Conditioning Exercises."

15. Abdomen Injuries and Care

General Discussion

The abdomen encompases a large area mostly below the sternum. It is subdivided into many regions or quadrants divided from each other from the anterior midline intersecting perpendicularly a horizontal line passing through the umbilicus. Thus, using the above intersecting lines, we can identify the area, in case of injury, as the upper right or left quadrants or the lower left or right quadrants. Another commonly used term for this area is "epigastrium" or "epigastric region," referring to the area below the sternum and between the two coastal arches. The area of the abdomen most commonly injured is the abdominal wall. The abdominal wall points out from the anterolateral (front and side) abdominal muscles of the lumbar area and points out from the muscles of the lower ribs and the diaphragm.

All abdominal injuries must be considered serious especially if there is a history of direct blow or fall to a hard surface. Once fracture has been ruled out, then we must proceed to treat this injury according to the diagnosis given by the physician or the hospital emergency care.

Signs and Symptoms

1. Swelling
2. Pain
3. Rigidity of injured area
4. Vomiting
5. Pallor
6. High pulse rate
7. Shock
8. Knees pulled up toward the chest
9. Chills

10. Sweating
11. Palpation tenderness
12. Collapse

The above signs and symptoms don't necessarily occur in every injury of the abdominal wall. All of the abdominal injuries combined, however, will present most of the above signs and symptoms.

Contusions

Abdominal contusion is the result of a direct blow to the abdominal wall, causing damage to the underlying tissues without breaking the overlying skin.

Signs and Symptoms

1. Pain
2. Rigidity
3. Vomiting (sometimes, depending on the degree and strength of the blow)
4. Pallor
5. Shock
6. Knees pulled up toward the chest

Immediate treatment

1. Ice-pack applications.
2. Abdominal strapping (Figure 71) or abdominal binder (commercially available).
3. Emergency care at the hospital to rule out internal injury.

Follow-up Care (after second or third day)

1. Application of heat (moist heat preferable).
2. Mild exercise. (If coughing produces a lot of pain, active exercise should be limited.)
3. Active abdominal exercises.
4. Progressive resistive exercises of abdominals. (See specific abdominal exercises in the last chapter of the book entitled "General Conditioning Exercise.")

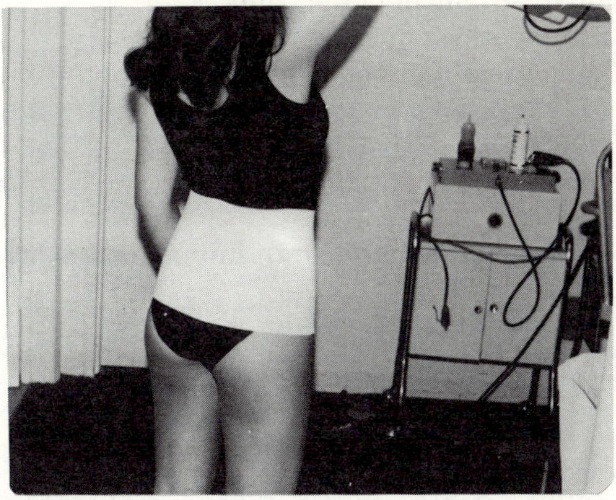

Figure 71. Abdominal strapping or abdominal binder (commercially available); also to be used for low back injury.

5. Flexible casting should be applied upon completion of treatment and during mild field workout.

6. Light field workout should begin at the end of the week after injury.

Note: The injured athlete should be the one to make the decision concerning his return to play. He should keep in mind that an early participation might impede the healing process of his injury and further his disability. At the same time, an overcautious and an overprotective athlete will retard his level of performance due to his prolonged absence from the game.

Ruptured Obliques

A ruptured oblique is any tear of any of its fibers along its continuity either from the point of origin or from its insertion. It occurs usually from a sudden twisting or due to a direct heavy blow to a tense muscle.

Signs and Symptoms

1. Localized pain.
2. Pain during any movement of the abdominal wall, as in sneezing, coughing, or in bowel movement.

3. Limited movement of the trunk.
4. Local tenderness during palpation.
5. Bulging areas occasionally.

Treatment (Immediately after injury)

1. Application of ice packs until inflammation subsides.
2. Flexible cast.

Follow-up Treatment—After 2nd or 3rd day

1. Moist heat for 20–30 minutes.
2. Massage (effleurage) around the injured area.
3. Medcoallator (pulsating mild electrical currents).
4. Manual muscle reeducation for optimum muscle strength.

Note: Any abdominal injury, whether a rupture, strain, or contusion, at times may produce low-back pain and discomfort. The anterior abdominal musculature plays a major role in maintaining the "anatomical corset" along with the glutei muscles by providing support to the lumbosacral spine. Consequently, any imbalance of this protective "corset" will produce repercussion to the low back. Therefore, during abdominal injuries, the treatment rationale should extend to the low back as well by applying moist heat and mild isometric exercises to the glutei, especially the gluteus maximus, bilaterally. Isometric exercises to pain tolerance should also be applied to the abdominals. Mild low-back exercises as described in an earlier chapter should be applied when preceded by heat applications. Not all abdominal injuries have low-back repercussions. In the few injuries where low back pain is produced, the above treatment is recommended not only for eliminating the low back discomfort, but also for the enhancement of the healing process of the abdominal injury.

Ruptured Rectus Abdominis

Any tear in the continuity of this muscle is considered to be a rupture. The same applies to injuries of the rectus abdominis, which very seldom occurs in well-trained athletes. The function of the rectus abdominis is to flex the trunk by bringing the xiphoid process of the sternum toward the pubic symphysis. The rectus abdominis serves the abdomen anteriorly as an elastic corset to support the abdominal viscera and, in view of its attachments anteriorly, plays a major role in the movements of the trunk. Although the role of this muscle is not one of mobility, it is directly related to the overall stability of the player. A player with poorly conditioned rectus abdominis will function very sluggishly and will be prone to injury as opposed to a well-conditioned muscle.

There are many ways of strengthening this muscle, although it is very difficult to isolate it from the rest of the abdominals. Situps with knees bent and feet flat on the floor are the most popular method for strengthening this muscle. (Figure 72) There are many versions of situps for the upper muscle fibers as well as the lower muscle fibers of the rectus abdominis. A more detailed exercise program will be discussed in the later chapter entitled "General Conditioning Exercises."

Immediate and Aftercare

Immediate and aftercare of a ruptured rectus abdominis does not differ from the treatment for ruptured obliques. Keep in mind that first

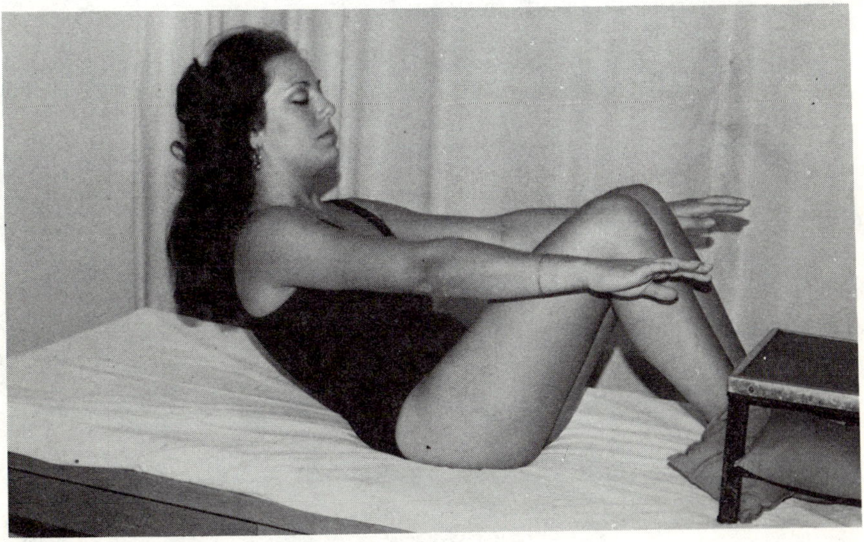

(a)

Figure 72. Sit-ups, progressive steps a, b, c, d.

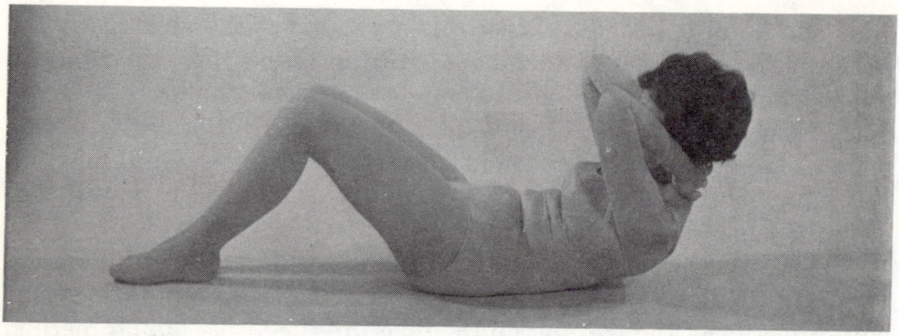

(b)

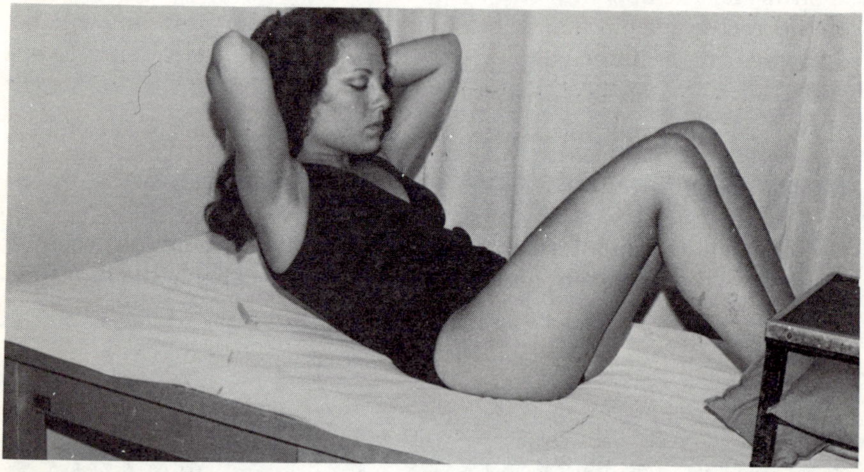

(c)

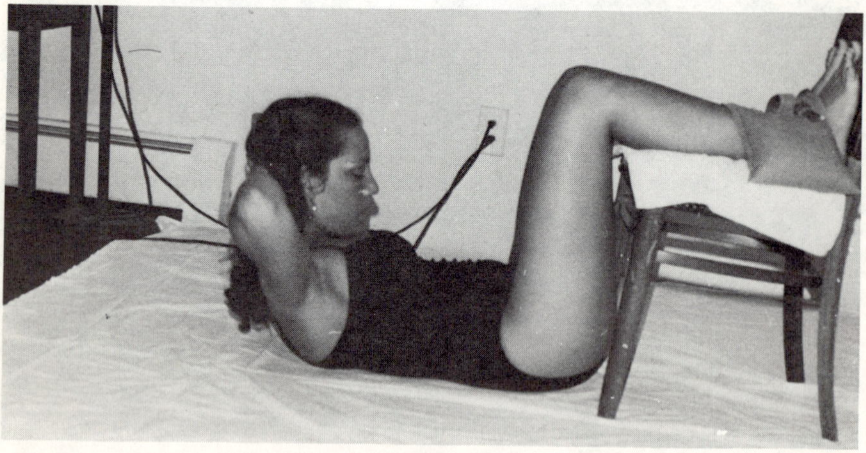

(d)

aid is always the most critical part of the therapeutic program. The application of an ice pack and the abdominal binder should always be available. The rehabilitation techniques should be applied immediately after the pain subsides without any further delay. A well-trained athlete recuperates much faster after a ruptured muscle. In view of the formation of the rectus abdominis into divided segments, this injury very rarely necessitates surgery after a rupture. In general, the ruptured fibers are so small that surgery is not even considered.

Abdominal Rigidity

This is a term usually applied in athletics. This discussion will only be applied to athletes and their injuries. It is not a symptom of disease and is defined as "the extreme tension of abdominal muscles over an area of localized tenderness or irritation." The most common causes of abdominal rigidity are:

1. Inadequate conditioning
2. Direct blow to the abdomen
3. Poor training
4. Appendicitis

Signs and Symptoms

1. Localized rigidity according to area involved.
2. Extremely painful contracted abdominal muscles.
3. Tachycardia (fast pulse).
4. Sweating.
5. Chills.
6. Collapse.

Treatment

1. Application of cold packs to the area.
2. History of trauma.
3. Emergency care is cold packs to relieve the pain and discomfort.
4. Preconditioning program of progressive resistive exercises for untrained athletes.
5. Keep players active when not performing, especially during cold-weather conditions.

6. Acclimatization of players with extra sessions of warmups when traveling to cold climates.

7. Adjustment periods for acclimatization between 12 and 48 hours.

Note: Superficial abdominal injuries repair quickly through periods of bed rest. Rigidity signs in muscles disappear within 24 hours. In deep abdominal injuries where the pulse gets much weaker and the athlete becomes pale and weak, emergency medical care is of the utmost importance.

16. Head and Neck Injuries and Care

General Discussion (Figures 73a–73e)

Severe head and neck injuries very seldom occur among soccer players. In those rare cases, a number of significant observations must be made in order to ensure the player's safety and in order to evaluate the player's condition. The head and neck comprise the most vital parts of the human body such as: the brain, the facial structures (eyes, ears, nose, mouth), the spinal cord, nerve roots, and vascular channels. Every head injury is complicated by the loss of oxygen to the brain, which, under severe conditions, might cause death. Neck injuries may bring radiating pain to shoulder and upper extremities, characterized by numbness, tingling, lack of sensation, and even loss of function when the nerve roots or spinal cord are involved. In these types of injuries, the player should be removed by stretcher and sent immediately to the hospital for emergency care, further tests, and observations.

Signs and Symptoms

1. Dazed momentarily.
2. Experiencing momentary unconsciousness.
3. Shaking his head to eliminate dizziness.
4. Difficulty or inability opening and closing the eyelids.

Note: At times, the player is collapsing on the floor, and the trainers apply a stick of aromatic ammonia under the athlete's nose. If the injury is not determined, and the athlete is lying down, *DO NOT* introduce sniffing ammonia because the sudden movement of the head from sniffing might worsen the condition.

5. Wobbly knees or rubbery legs.
6. Glassy eyes with fixed glazed stare.

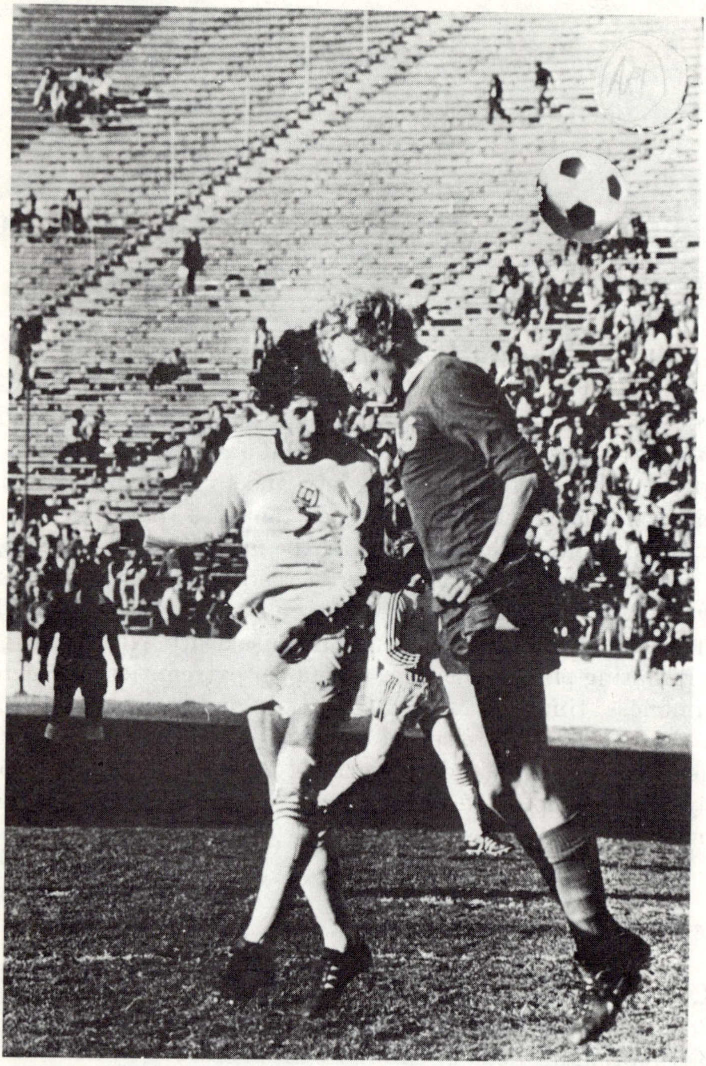

Figure 73a. Head collision with possible concussion.

7. Pupils: fixed, dilated, or unequal (warning for immediate removal from the game and into emergency care).

Note: In case of sustained muscular tension (tonic contractions) or alternating contraction and relaxation (clonic contractions) of the muscles of the face, neck, trunk, and the extremities ending in con-

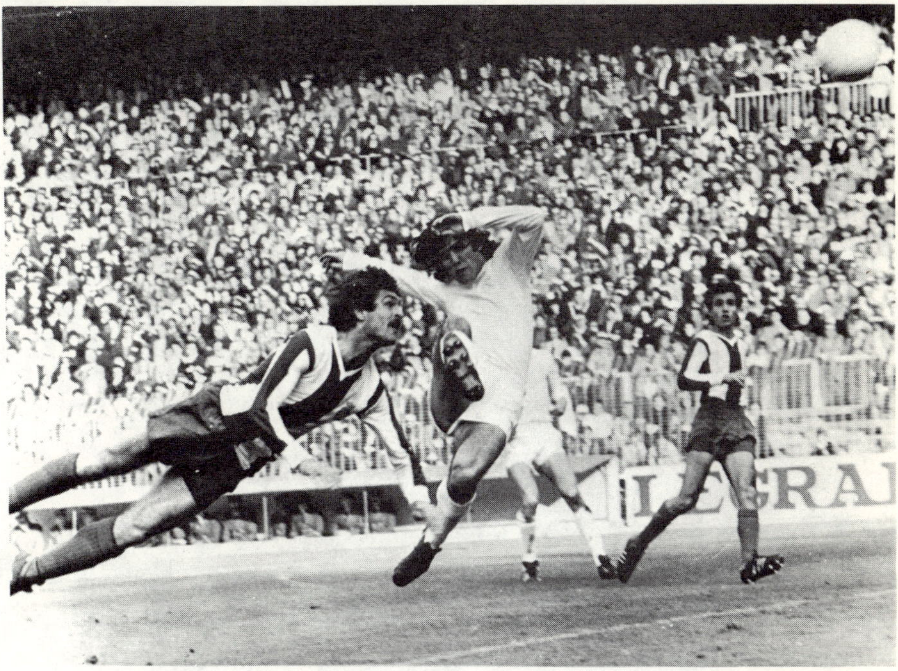

Figure 73b. Head and neck injuries.

vulsive movements, the removal of the player from the game on a stretcher is indicated. The player's head during such injuries should be placed on one side with support to the chin, thus preventing the tongue from being swallowed. Also, this position allows the saliva to run out. Any form, however minimal, of bleeding from the ear indicates immediate emergency hospital care.

Neck Injuries: Signs and Symptoms

1. Pain and numbness down to the arm, hand, or both
2. Weakness of one or both hands
3. Dizziness
4. Momentarily incoherent
5. At times unconscious
6. Pain and/or spasm of the anterior and posterior neck muscles
7. Limited R.O.M. (range of motion)

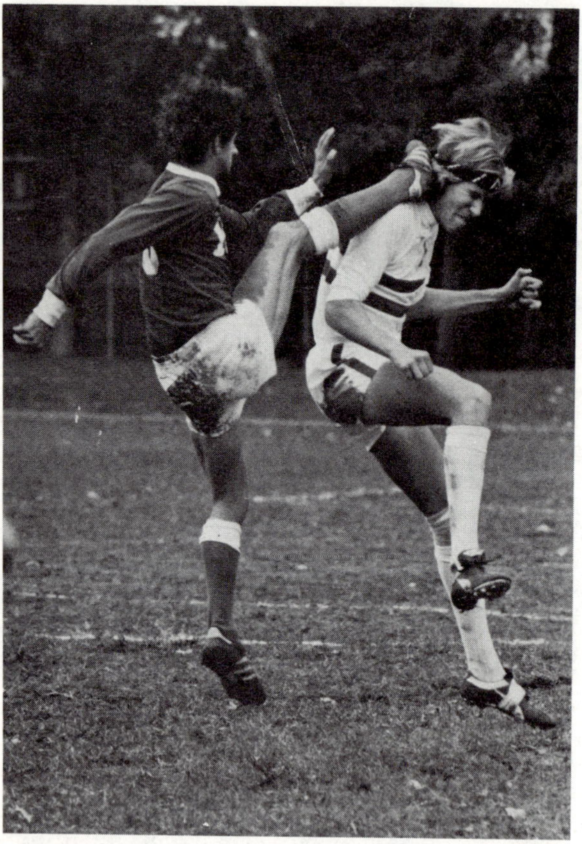

Figure 73c. Neck injuries involving the face.

Immediate Care

In minor injuries of the neck not accompanied by head injuries, the player may be allowed to return to the game provided no neurological signs are present (numbness, weakness, pain) and the range of motion of the neck is normal. In head injuries, when any of the above signs and symptoms are present, do not move nor manipulate the player's head. If the injured player is coherent and can follow instructions, get a full history of the injury. Observe any obvious abnormalities and any limitations of movement. Have athlete sit comfortably and wait for physician's instructions. In neck injuries, the same procedure should be applied, emphasizing stabilization of the

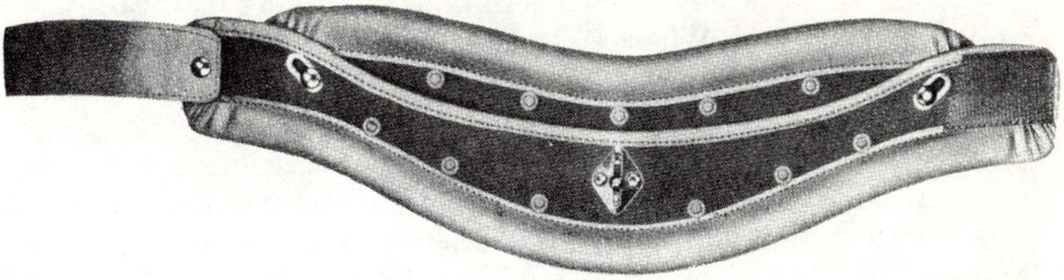

Figure 73. Cervical collar, adjutable (Courtesy of Geremi Surgicals).

head and neck with sandbags or foam cushion positioners. If active movement of the neck is present, remove the athlete off the field with a stretcher. The best care of neck injuries is prevention. Prevention, through preseason calisthenics to develop strength for anterior and posterior neck muscles as well as shoulder muscles is the best method of eliminating 95 percent of possible neck injuries. When repeated neck injuries occur resulting in calcifications (calcium deposits) between the vertebrae of the neck, then other methods, designed to eliminate restruction in R.O.M., prevent atrophy of disuse, and increase muscle strength to the muscles surrounding the cervical spine (neck), must be employed. Thus, the following physical therapy program should be instituted:

1. Moist heat for 20 minutes.
2. Cervical traction intermittently (preferable to constant traction).
3. Medcosonlator to neck and shoulder muscles (assist in reducing muscle spasm and reduce pain).
4. Active R.O.M. of the neck.
5. Manual resistive exercises in all directions.
6. Cervical collar, (Figure 73) in slight neck flexion preventing hyperextension of the neck (commercially available).

Note: Physical therapy plays an important role mostly in prevention of neck injuries. A preseason strengthening exercise program emphasizing exercises to such groups of muscles as the neck flexors (sternocleidomastoids) as well as the neck extensors (upper trapezii) will serve as an important means of prevention.

Concussion

Any blow to the head may cause a concussion. The degree (mild or severe) of concussion is dependent on the athlete's maintaining his intellectual faculties. Where the athlete receives a blow and is knocked out momentarily, regaining his consciousness immediately, then he has suffered a mild concussion. Where the athlete's unconsciousness extends over a minute along with headache, dizziness, and loss of intellect, then he has suffered a severe concussion. The longer the recovery time, the more severe the damage to the brain. If any of the later symptoms are evident, the athlete should be moved by stretcher off the playing area and into the hospital where the services of a neurosurgeon will be indicated. If a player's unconsciousness extends for more than a minute, it should be a routine practice to have the player hospitalized under observation for twenty-four hours.

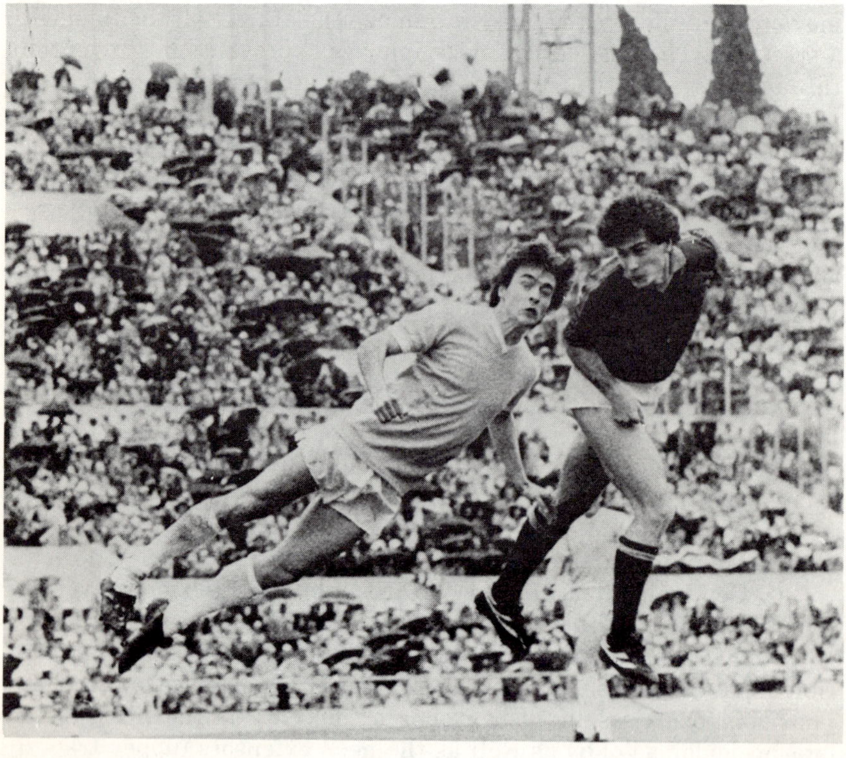

Figure 73d. Head, neck, and shoulder injuries.

Mild Concussion

Before the player is permitted to return to the game he must:

1. Not complain of headache
2. Not complain of dizziness
3. Be fully conscious

Severe Concussion

1. The player must not return to the game; no school spirit or team spirit should persuade the player to return.

2. The player must be evaluated by a physician, possibly a neurosurgeon, and be evaluated periodically.

3. He should not participate in any activity for at least 2 weeks, after which he should consult his physician for further evaluation.

Questions to be asked when testing player's faculties

1. Your name?
2. Your address?
3. Attending school?
4. Where are you now?
5. What is your profession?
6. What is the name of your team?
7. Do you see double?
8. Can you open and close your eyes?
9. Can you follow my finger with your eyes?
10. Lift your hand up.
11. Squeeze my hand.
12. Whistle by placing lips together and blow.

Note: The trainer must keep a record of all head injuries whether mild or severe, which might be very effective in establishing a diagnosis and the future care of the athlete.

Torn Neck Muscles

The history of the injury as well as the visual signs followed by the player's description will enhance the evaluation and make the handling much easier. When fractures have been ruled out, the following procedures should be applied:

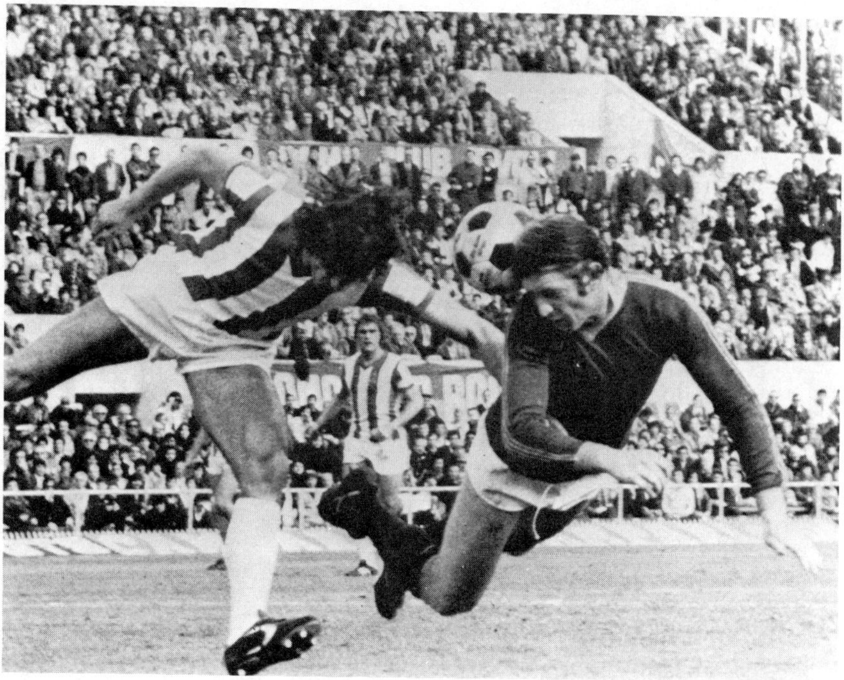

Figure 73e. Head and upper trunk injuries.

1. The use of a collar (made out of a foam rubber with velcro straps).

2. Ice pack applications for the first 24 hours.

3. Massage in the form of effleurage around the trapezius area (upper trapezius).

4. Intermittent traction after full range of motion has been completed—usually fourth or fifth day, starting with 12 pounds and progressively proceeding to 20 pounds or to pain tolerance.

5. Medcosonlator the fifth day as tolerated.

6. The use of the collar should extend to at least the first week after injury.

7. Progressive resistive exercises (P.R.E.) usually after complete R.O.M. has been attained.

8. P.R.E. to be applied in all areas of neck movement.

9. Continue heat massage and exercise three times daily.

Note: Disability in torn muscles of the neck varies between 5 days and 2 weeks, depending on the degree of tear and the muscles involved. The most common muscles that are usually torn are the upper and middle fibers of trapezius, which are the neck extensors, and the sternocleidomastoids, which are the neck flexors and rotators. However, never in my experience have I seen both injuries occur simultaneously. Usually, they tear individually whether from extreme neck rotation or from extreme lateral flexion (bending of the neck to respective shoulder).

Muscle Spasm

It is a warning of very tight muscles. This phenomenon should not be ignored because it will result in a torn muscle. Muscle spasm usually occurs after an injury such as a pulled muscle, a torn muscle, or a contusion. The spasm is a warning that indicates that if the injury is not treated immediately, more muscle fibers will be torn. Muscle spasm usually occurs in the back of the neck and at the lumbosacral area (low-back area). The treatment of muscle spasm depends on the number of fibers torn: whether a few fibers or the rupture of many. Ice-pack applications for the first 24 hours bring relief and reduce the disability. The application of Medcosonlator to trigger points is also very helpful. Finally, mild intermittent traction preceded by moist heat has reportedly been used very successfully in treating muscle spasms in the posterior cervical spine (back of the neck). If muscle spasms are not recognized immediately and are not treated properly, they can be a real pain in the neck.

PART III
TRAINING ROOM EQUIPMENT AND SUPPLIES

GENERAL DISCUSSION

The training room ideally should be separated from the dressing room and should be available to all soccer players. This room should be somewhat special, creating a special therapeutic atmosphere. The room should be cheerfully lighted and well ventilated. In view of the electrical equipment used for injuries, it should have enough electrical outlets and adequate voltage for excessive use when necessary. The water pressure should be adequate, as should water drains, for the use of at least two whirlpools. Wall cabinets for linen, refrigerator for ice making, and storage for sterile dressings should be standard equipment. Desk, filing cabinet for records, treatment tables, benches, and chairs should be part of the training-room equipment. Other necessary equipment will be discussed later.

17. First-Aid Kit

First-aid kits are very useful and must be carried on the soccer field or on away games. Whether the team plays on a home field or away, this first-aid kit must be on the grounds at all times. Often, the first-aid kit might save a player's life and/or might lessen the extent of disability. The contents of a first-aid kit are usually those requested by the trainer. Most of the contents are usually found in surgical and sport supply stores. The first-aid kit that I highly recommend is one that was given to us by a surgical and sport supply company in Astoria, N.Y., namely, Geremi Surgical And Sport Supply, Inc. The most important first-aid kit equipment will be outlined, underlined, and described below.

Scissors: Necessary for removing clothing fast and effectively as well as for cutting and applying taping.

Eye Cup: Necessary for eye washing, removing dirt, etc.

Sling: Usually for immobilizing shoulder injuries.

Alcohol: To be used as an antiseptic or for light massage.

Skin Toughener: Can be purchased under the name tincture of benzoin and can be used before taping with adhesive powder.

Powder: Can be used as a massage agent and also after taping to avoid sticking to clothing.

Spirits of Ammonia: To be used carefully for restoring unconscious athletes.

Aspirin: For relief of pregame headaches of players and/or other members of the coaching staff.

Tongue depressors: For possible seizures or to be used for splinting injuries of the fingers.

Oral Screw: To be used for lockjaw during a seizure.

Flexible Casting: Necessary for strapping in injuries of arms and legs.

Elastic Bandaging: Necessary for wrapping injuries of arms and legs of minor nature.

Dressing: Any material applied to any part of the body for protection, stimulation, repair, and drain with or without the carrying of medicated solutions.

—*Dry*—to be used in sterile form for punctured wounds with drugs (ointments or powder) and without drugs. Example, Telfa Pads are sterile and can be used with drugs and without them. They are made with a nonsticky element.

—*Moist*—Those that provide local hyperemia, saturated with prescribed solutions. They are also sterile.

Ice Packs: To be used for sprains, strains, or contusions by providing immediate local cold.

Splints: Air splints are plastic air bags that can be blown by mouth after the involved injured extremity (arm or leg) has been inserted in the bag. They are very popular because of their practical and safe use. They come in all sizes and can be used for severe sprains, for questionable fractures or other severe arm or leg injuries. They are used mostly prior to emergency hospital care for x-rays and/or other examinations.

Standard splints are made out of wood or plastic boards that are wrapped around the injured part before the athlete is taken to emergency care in the hospital. They are known as Jordan splints.

18. Training Room

Training-room equipment must fulfill the needs of all injuries sustained during the soccer season. A very careful study by the team physician, the physical therapist, and the trainer of the injuries sustained in the past (at least the past three years) will establish a pretty good idea in the basics of training-room equipment. The most standard training-room equipment, which will fulfill most of the needs of any soccer team, will be outlined, underlined, and described below as follows:

Treatment Table: It can be used for massage, therapeutic exercise, taping and other essential uses. A standard table should be 6 feet long, 2 feet wide, and 3 feet high.

Stretcher: A folding adjustable with wheels (6-inch diameter), which can be changed to a chair and/or to a stretcher, depending on the particular need. It should be used for transporting injured players to the ambulance or to emergency hospital care.

Blankets: Always useful during the winter season for keeping the injured player warm.

Liniment: Necessary for prewarmup massage, usually for the older players during cold winter games. In my opinion, pregame calisthenics, in the form of stretching and general conditioning, is the best pregame warmup. Liniments are commercially available in drug stores and in some sport-supplies stores. However, each trainer has his own formula. One formula that I recommend is a mixture of 6 parts of Albalene cream to 2 parts of wintergreen. It is very inexpensive, easy to make, and very effective for pregame warmup massage.

Tape Remover: It comes in spray cans of 8 ounces, and it is very effective in reducing pain during removal of adhesive tape.

Antiseptic Soap: It should be present over the training room's sink and should be used constantly by the trainer when caring for superficial wounds.

Moleskin: It is smooth self-adhesive on one surface and smooth like velvet on the other surface. It has been used for splinting arms or legs.

Electric Hair Clipper: Very necessary for the care of superficial head wounds.

Gauze Pads: Come in all sizes and can be used for strapping and to hold dressings.

Medico Paste or "Una Boot": For sprains and strains.

Ortho-Plast Material: Excellent for splinting.

Plaster of Paris: For severe sprains or questionable fractures.

Adjustable Crutches: For leg injuries when weight bearing of the injured leg is not desirable or questionable. Usually, an adult adjustable crutch fits all adult sizes. The same thing in child's size applies to children.

Oral and Rectal Thermometers: Should be always available and used when in doubt about player's general condition.

Physical Therapy Equipment: Should be used under a registered physical therapist's supervision. The most desirable equipment to be found in training rooms is listed below:

1. Hydrocollator hot packs*
2. Whirlpools—stationary or portable for extremities or full body immersion*
3. Ultrasonics*
4. Heating lamps*
5. Ultraviolet machine
6. Medcollator
7. Medcosonlator
8. Transcutaneous electrical nerve stimulation
9. Short-wave diathermy
10. Paraffin tank
11. Quadriceps table (N/K Table)*
12. Adjustable resistance, bicycle

All training rooms must have the phone numbers of the nearest emergency hospitals conspicuously displayed on the desk or taped on the bulletin board. The same phone numbers should also be taped inside the first-aid kit.

*Necessary equipment for a low budget.

PART IV
GENERAL CONDITIONING EXERCISES

General Discussion

This part will present group exercises for all parts of the body. It will reinforce the previously mentioned exercises after injury. These exercises will be performed by the soccer player during practice sessions or on pregame warmups (calisthenics). The exercises may also be applied after an injury when exercise is permissible. A description in detail of each movement would result in very monotonous reading. The author of this book, therefore, decided to use live demonstrations represented by photos and illustrations. The reader consequently will have a better representation, and he or she will be able to assimilate the principles involved. General conditioning exercises will be divided into two different stages. The first stage will emphasize the active range of motion and its completion. Stretching and strengthening exercises (which represent the second stage) should not be attempted until the first stage is completed. Both stages will be very valuable from the therapeutic view point and very informative as well. Therapeutically, they will increase the range of movement when attempted repetitiously, and, consequently, when resistance is added, once complete range of motion has been reached, they will increase the strength. During the first stage, the player, when looking at the illustrations, will be learning and performing the possible approximate ranges of the joints of his body, which should be very constructive and informative.

19. Active Exercises for R.O.M.

Shoulder Exercises

1. Pendulum swinging—start with body in standing position semi-flexed. Swing arms forward and backward as shown, Figure 74.

2. Pendulum swinging—proceed the same with body from the waist up parallel with the floor, as shown. Proceed the same holding two pound barbell weight, Figure 75a, b, c.

3. Bringing arms behind back—bring injured arm behind with the assistance of the good arm. Proceed the same without any assistance. When complete R.O.M., use graded weights.

4. Bringing arm overhead—bring arm overhead with assistance. Assistance allowed only if the injured shoulder can not complete the movement. Proceed the same without assistance. When complete R.O.M., use graded weights under supervision.

5. Climbing wall with fingers—keep position of body straight while fingers are climbing the wall.

Note: When weights are being used, follow your physical therapist's instructions.

Neck Exercises

1. Lie flat on bed, fingers locked behind head. Use tension. Bring arms forward till forearms are touching sides of head.

2. Extend neck as far as possible. Rotate head toward either shoulder.

3. Extend neck as far as possible. Put hands on back of head, elbows back. Push neck forward with hands and resist with neck. Push back with neck and resist with hands to starting position.

Shoulder Exercises

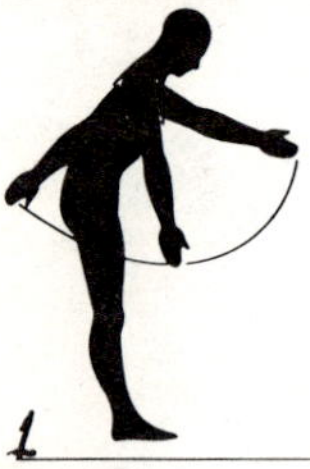

1.

1. Pendulum swinging

Start with body in standing position semi-flexed, swing arm forwards & backwards as illustrated.

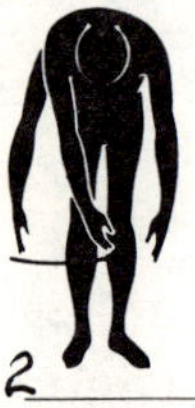

2.

2. Pendulum swinging

Proceed the same with body from the waist up parallel with the floor, as illustrated
Proceed the same holding 2 lbs of sandbag weight.

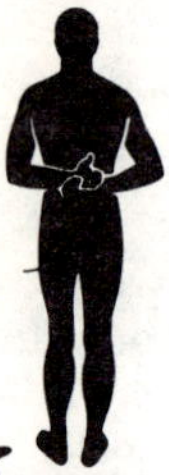

3.

3. Bringing arm behind back

bring injured arm behind with the assistance of the good arm.
proceed the same with any assistance.
when complete R.O.M. use graded wts.

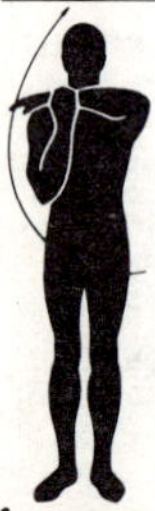

4.

4. Bringing arm overhead

bring arm overhead with assistance.
proceed the same with assistance
when complete R.O.M.; use graded wts. under supervision.

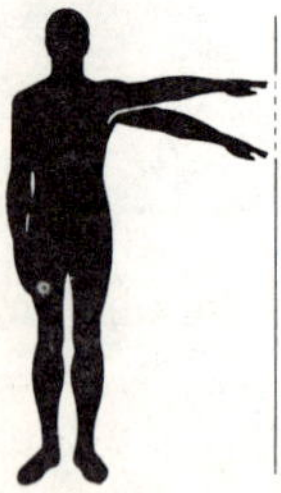

5.

5. Climbing wall with fingers

keep position of body straight while fingers are climbing the wall.

Note. when wts. are being used follow your physical therapists instructions.

Figure 74. Active exercise for R.O.M. Schematic representation of shoulder exercises. (Courtesy of Arthritis Foundation).

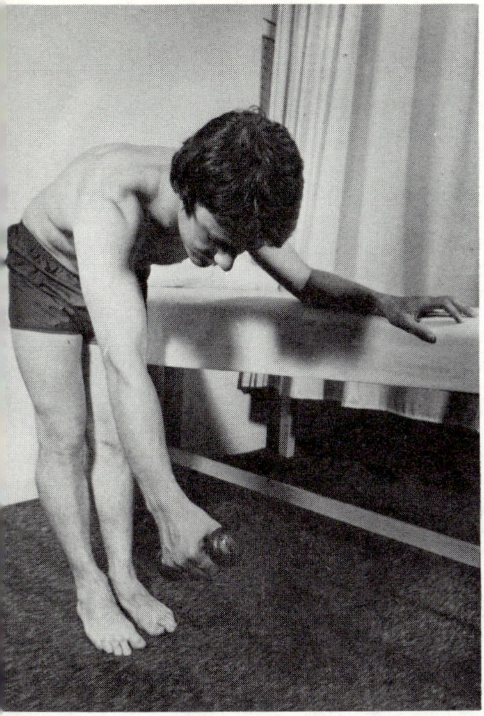

(a)

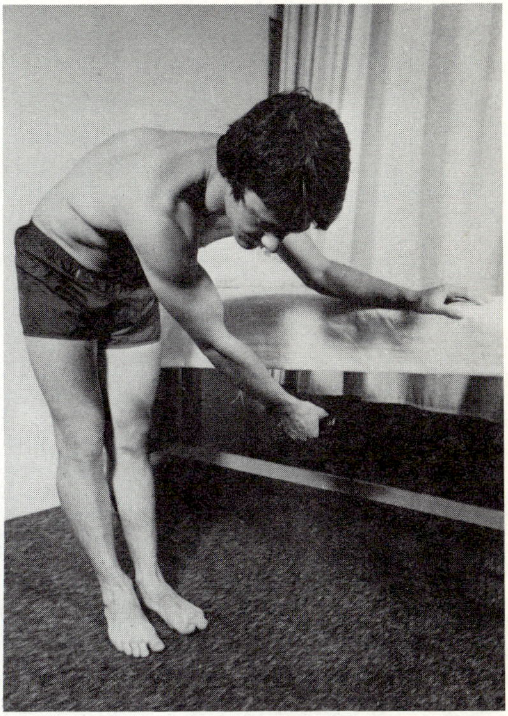

(c)

Figure 75a–c. Photographical representation of pendulum swinging exercises for treating shoulder stiffness.

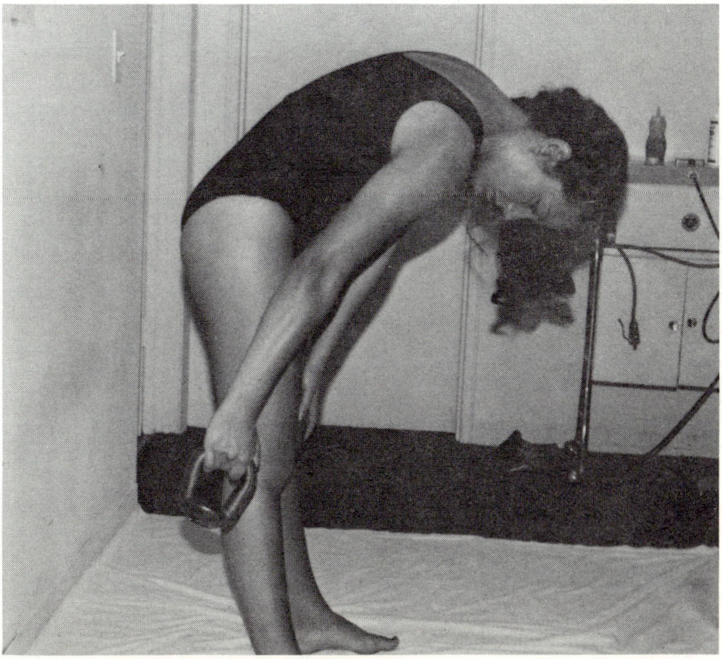

(b)

Back Exercises (Prevention of Back Pain) (Figure 76)

1. Rest position. Breathe deeply, raising chest. Exhale by drawing upper abdomen in. Take next breath against uplifted chest.

2. Tighten lower abdominal muscles. Relax.

3. Flatten back against floor by tightening lower abdomen and buttocks at the same time. Relax.

4. Hug both knees to chest.

5. Hug one knee to chest. Raise other leg straight and lower slowly, keeping abdomen in.

6. Lie in the prone position. Pillow under abdomen, tighten buttocks. Relax.

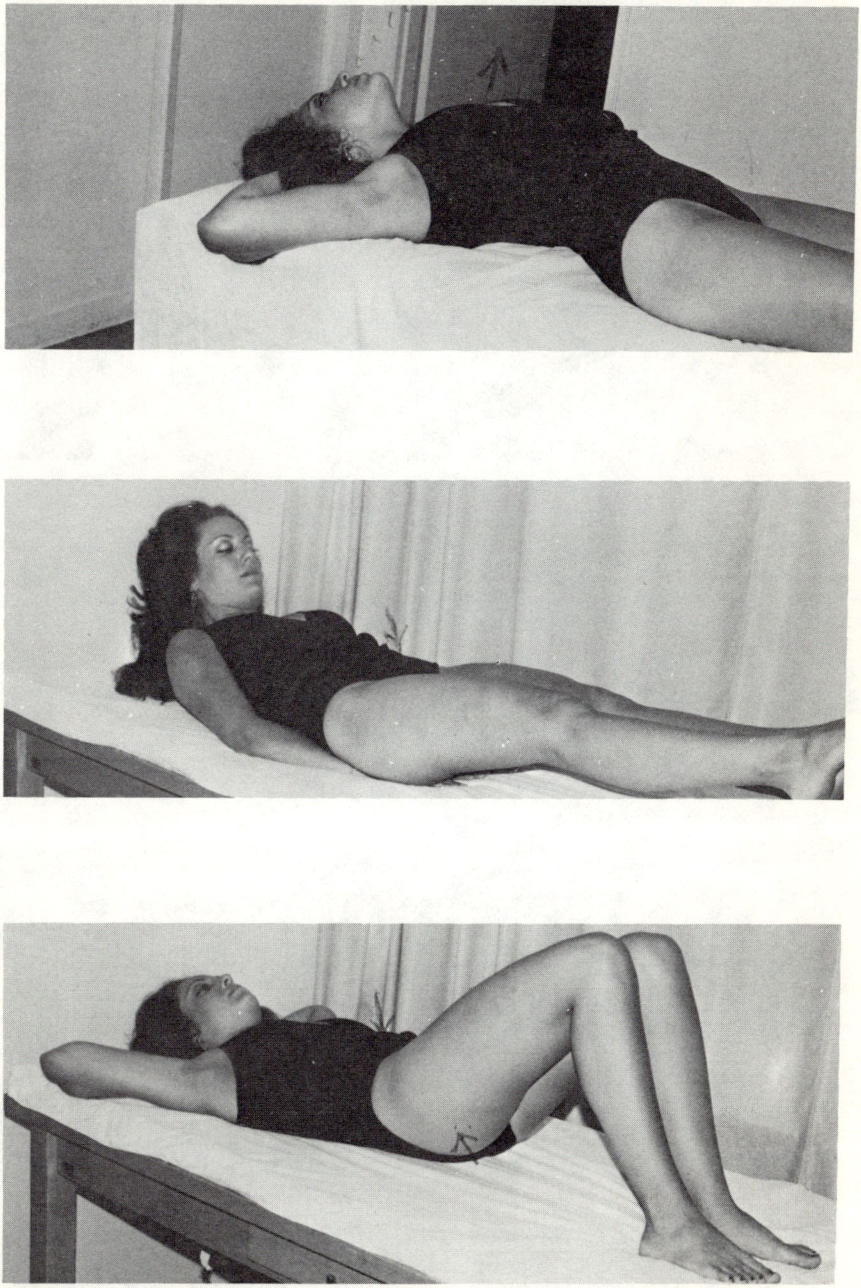

Figure 76. Back exercises—prevention of back pain.

Figure 76 (Continued)

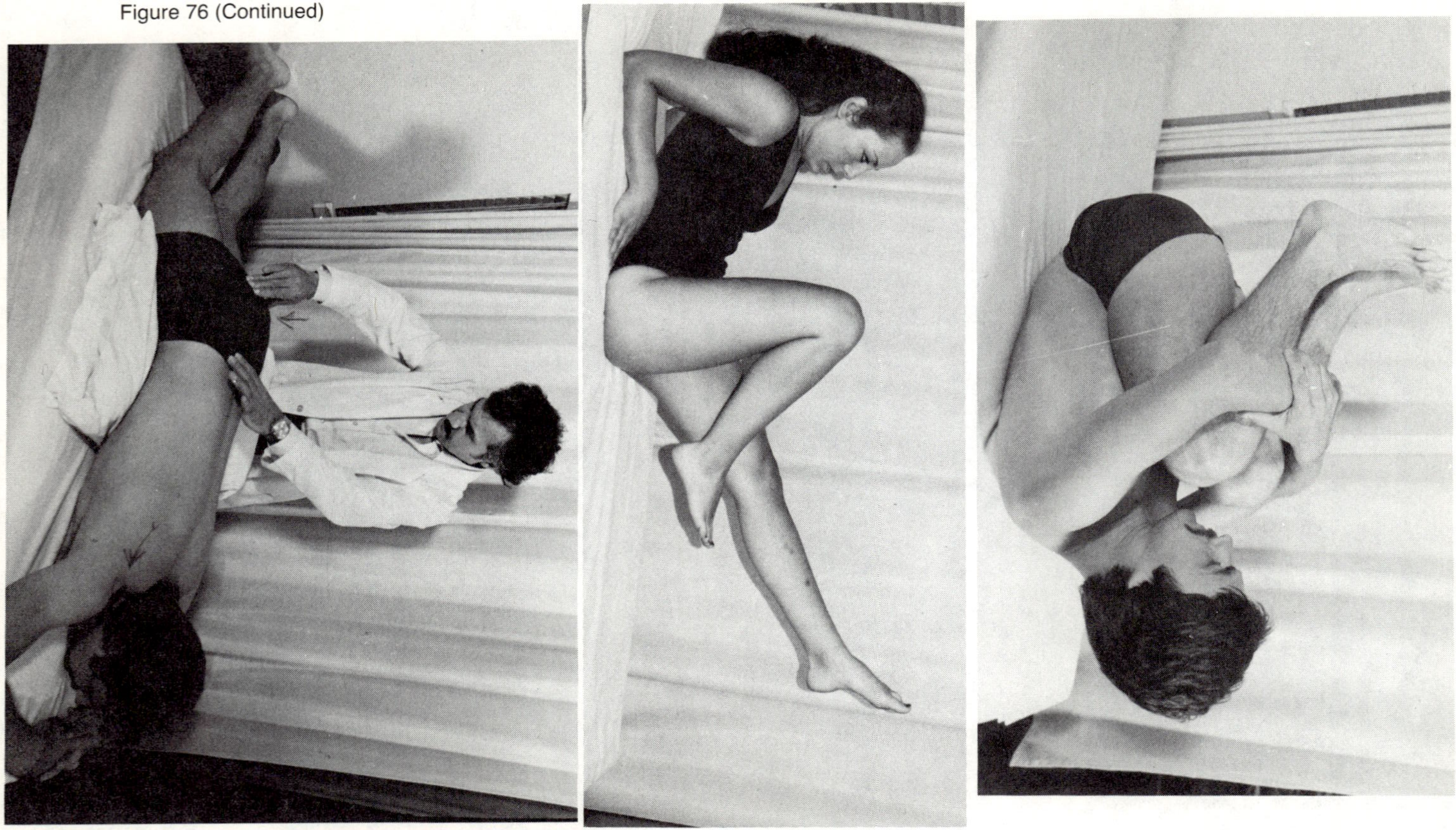

Hip and Knee Exercises

Figure 77. This exercise checks the rotary movements of the hip joints.

1. Hip rotation internally.
2. Hip rotation externally.
3. Straight leg raising: a self-applied test to check the tightness of the hamstrings.

Figure 78. Alternate Hip and Knee Exercises (Schematic Interpretation—Courtesy of Arthritis Foundation).

1. Lie flat on your back (supine) with your heels about 15 inches apart. Touch big toes to each other without inverting ankle. Then the opposite direction by rotating thighs externally.
2. Raise one leg to a right angle position with the trunk. Lower slowly. Alternate.
3. Flex thigh and raise to right angle with trunk. Extend lower leg straight with thigh. Lower slowly.
4. Legs straight. Tighten the abdominals and thigh muscles, relax and repeat. Do not lift your legs—only tighten muscles.
5. Lie on your stomach. Raise the leg with knee straight. Lower slowly. Note: Do not lift the pelvis, just the leg, straight upwards.
6. Lie on your stomach. Bend the lower leg and try to touch heel to buttocks. Proceed from above position to lift knee upwards. This exercise will strengthen your buttocks.

Hands, Feet, and Elbows Exercises (Figure 79)

1. *Wrist and forearm.* Grasp the handle of a medium-weight hammer firmly near its head. Turn your wrist from left to right and back. Let the weight of the hammer swing your hand over as far as possible each time. As you improve, shift your grip farther toward the end of the handle so that the weight of the hammer makes you work harder.
2. *Fingers and thumb.* Open and close your hands, spreading your fingers as you open them and making as tight a fist as possible when you close them. Touch the tip of your thumb to each finger in turn, pinching firmly each time. Try to form a letter "o" at each attempt.
3. *Ankle, for dorsiflexion.* Sit on a chair with your feet flat on the floor. Raise your toes as high as you can while keeping your heels down. (Maintain the upward position for six seconds or a slow count of six.)
4. *Ankle, for plantar flexion.* Repeat above by keeping your toes down and lifting your heels as high as possible.

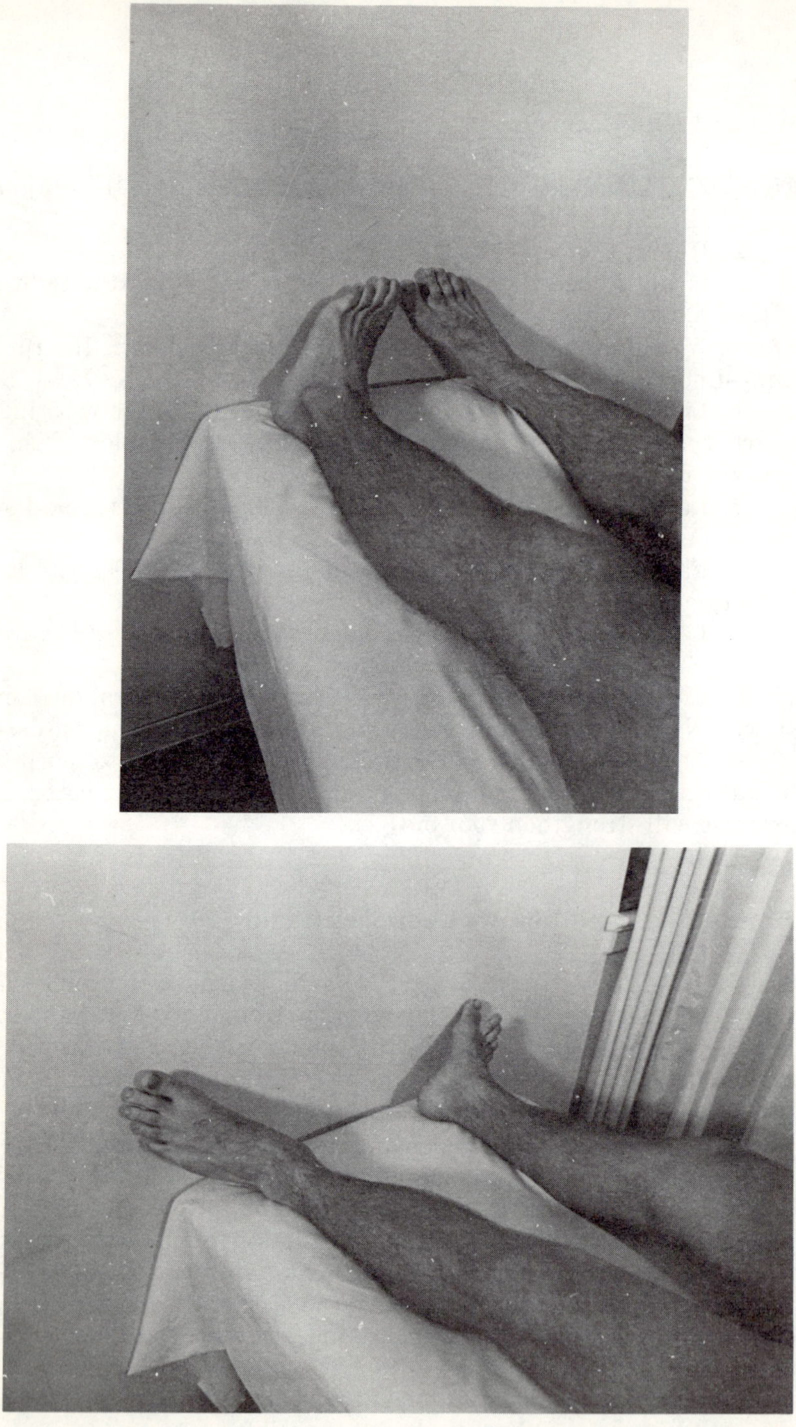

Figure 77. Hip and knee exercises (Photographic interpretation).

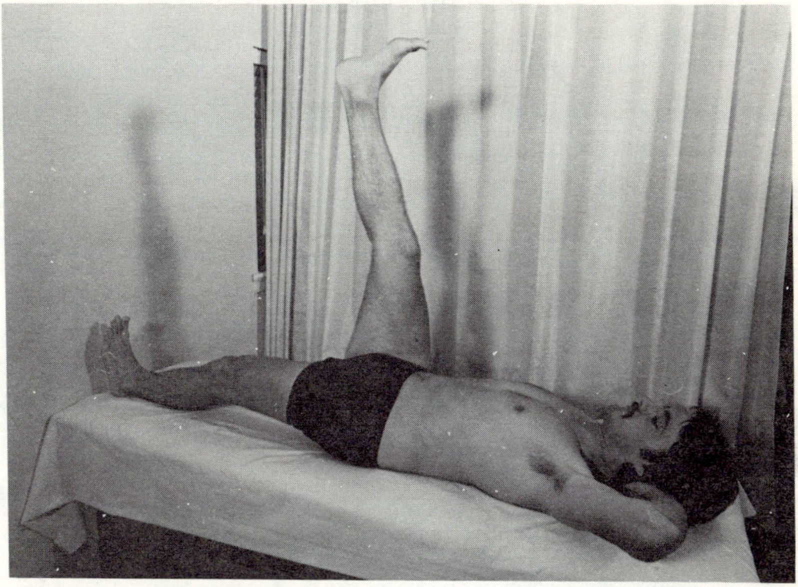

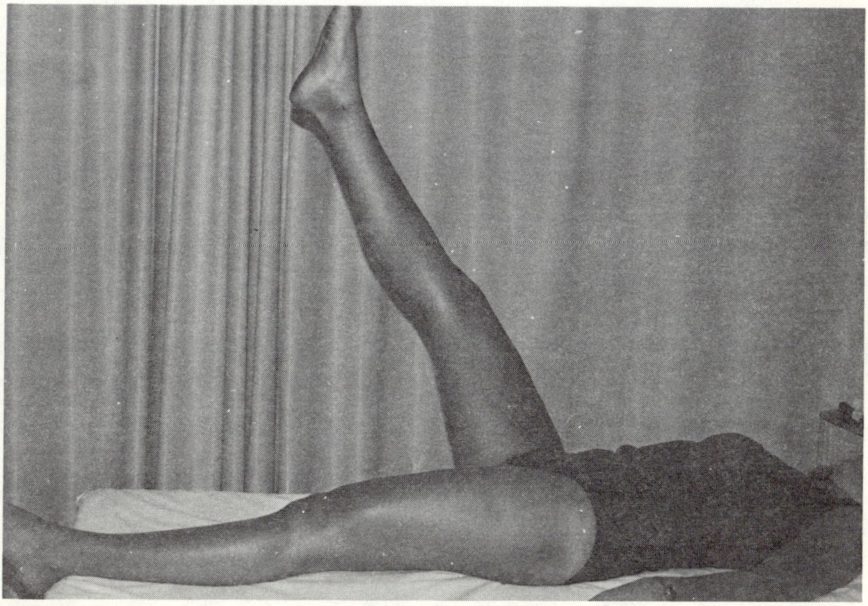

1. Lie flat on your back with your heels about 15 inches apart. Touch big toes to each other without inverting ankle. Then externally rotate thighs.

   This exercise when executed correctly with the knees straight and tight will promote rotary movements at the hip joint

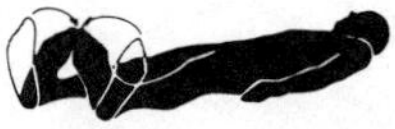

2. Raise one leg to a right angle position with the trunk. Lower slowly. Alternate.

   Do not force the movements.

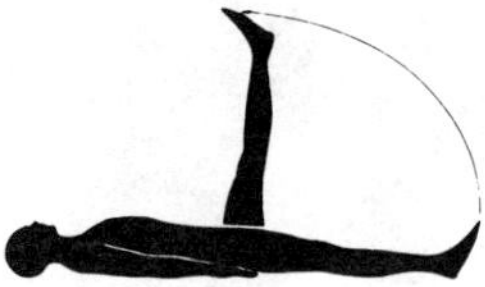

3. Flex thigh and raise to right angle with trunk. Extend lower leg straight with thigh. Lower slowly.

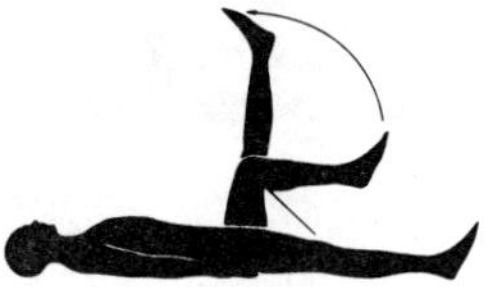

4. Leg straight. Tighten the thigh muscle, relax, repeat.

   NOTE: Do not lift your legs. Only tighten muscles

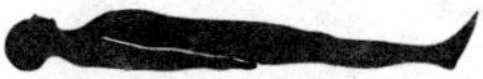

Figure 78. Alternate hip and knee exercises (Schematic interpretation Courtesy of Arthritis Foundation).

5. Lie on your stomach. Raise the leg with knee straight. Lower slowly.

Note. Do not lift the pelvis, just the leg, straight upwards.

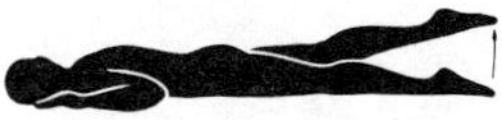

6. Lie on your stomach. Bend the lower leg and try to touch heel to buttocks.

Proceed from above position to lift knee upwards. This exercise will strengthen your buttocks.

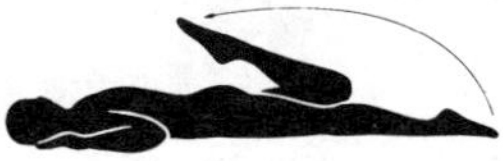

5. *Ankle, for inversion.* Same position. Lift the inside of each foot and roll the weight over the outside of the foot. Keep your toes curled down if possible.

6. *Ankle, for eversion.* Rotate the ankle in a circle, curling toes upward and downward.

7. *Shoulder and elbow in flexion abduction and rotation.* Touch your hand to your shoulder (same side) and return to the starting position (palm and thumb up).

8. *Shoulder and elbow in flexion.* Same as above with gradual weight increase.

9. *Wrist and shoulder isometrically performed.* Stand two to three feet from the wall, with arms reaching forward at shoulder level. Rest hands on wall and lean forward bending the elbows until the hands touch the shoulders.

Special note: All above exercises are simply preliminary exercises prior to the progressive resistive exercises. It should be understood by everyone that the above exercises are basic and will give us an idea whether the muscle and joint involved are able for any form of exercise. In case there is limitation of movement and/or stiffness, we will not proceed with any form of strengthening exercise before this limitation disappears. In the meantime, the above exercises must continue until the R.O.M. is completed and the stiffness has been eliminated.

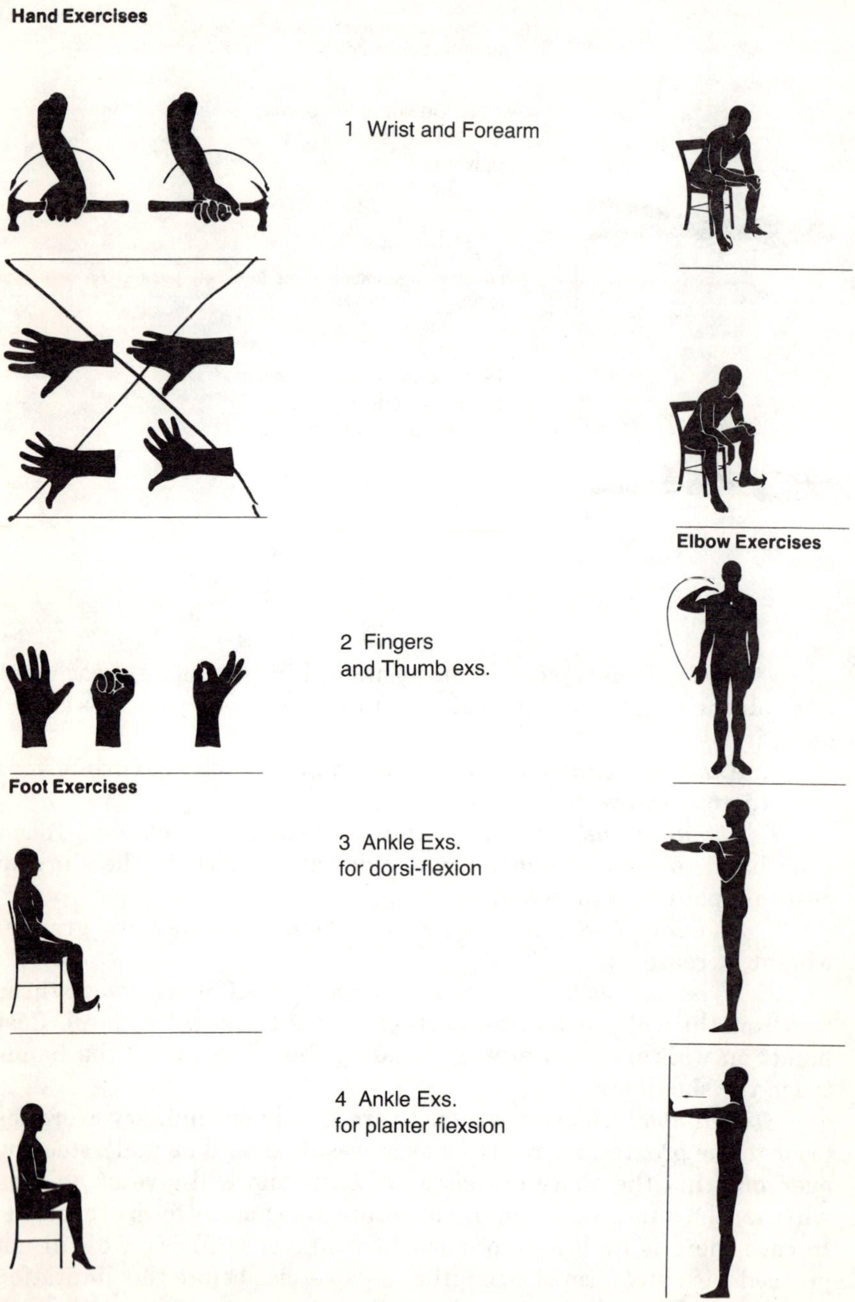

Figure 79. Hands, feet, and elbow exercises. Testing R.O.M. of elbow, forearm, wrist, hands, and feet. Active and resistive movements.

20. Stretching and Strengthening Exercises

These exercises strengthen the anterior, lateral, and medial muscles of the body.

Special Note: I would like to emphasize very strongly that the term stretching has been used in the form of self-stretching and *not* in the form of passive stretching which is administered to the injured player by someone else.

—stretching the back and leg muscles in the standing, lying supine position

—stretching and strengthening of the abdominal and hip flexors musculature (upper and lower)

—stretching and strengthening the lateral (side) and medial muscles of the body.

Figure 80. Anterior, Lateral and Medial Muscles of the Body

1. Stretching thoracic cavity, abdominals, and anterior shoulder musculature: breathing in and breathing out.
2. Stretching thigh and knee muscles: glutei, hamstrings, and, partially, gastrocnemius.

Figure 80A. Abdominal and Hip Flexors

3. Stretching above muscles from standing position.
4. Stretching above muscles from lying prone (on stomach).
5. Stretching back and leg muscles from standing position.
6. Stretching pectorals partially, and lumbo-sacral structures.
7. Strengthening upper abdominals (note position of knees and feet).
8. Strengthening lower abdominals.

1

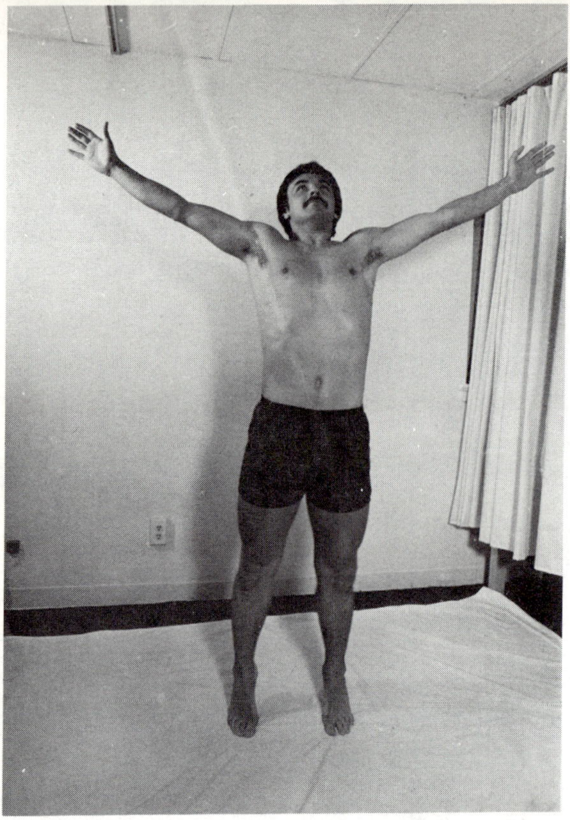

Figure 80. Stretching and strengthening exercises of the Anterior, Lateral, and Medial muscles of the body.

2

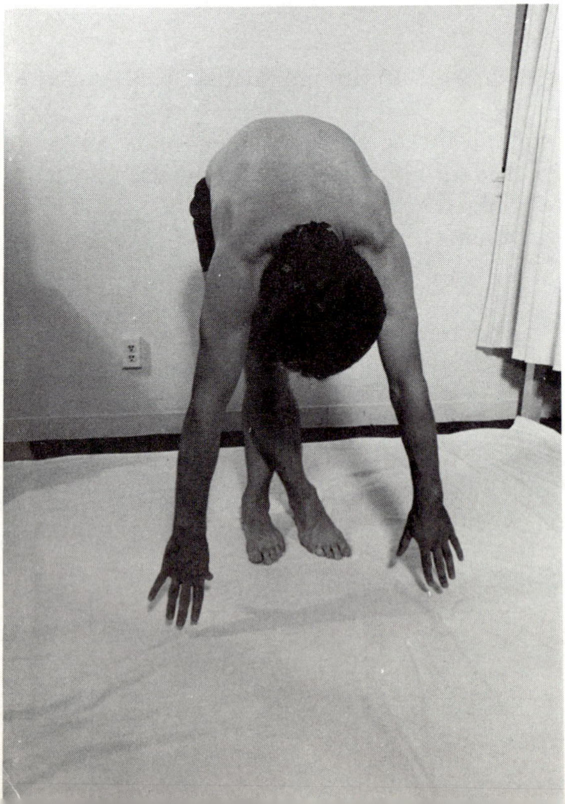

3

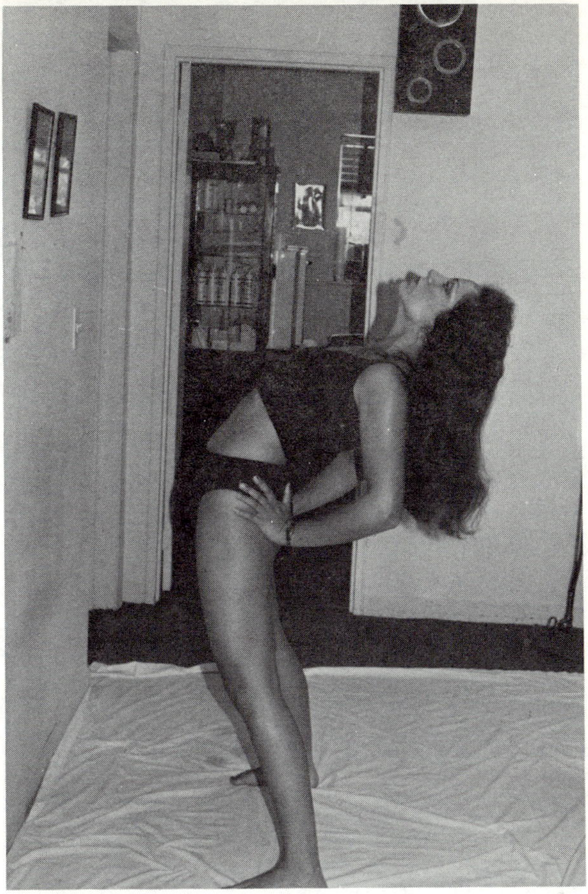

Figure 80a. Stretching abdominals and hip flexors

4

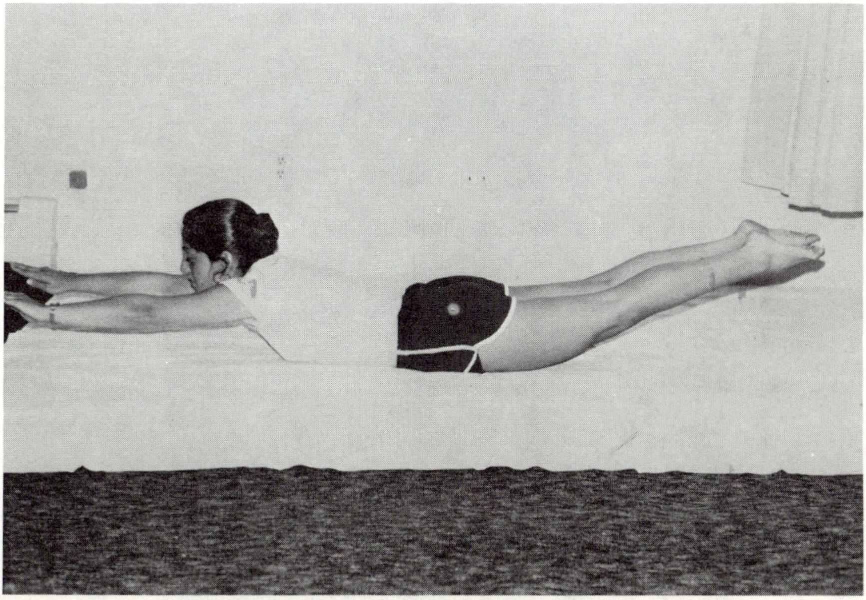

5

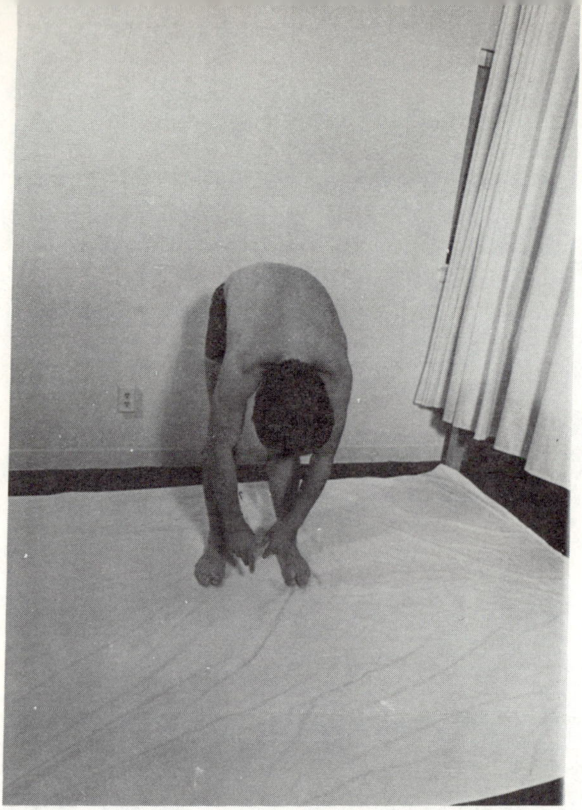

6

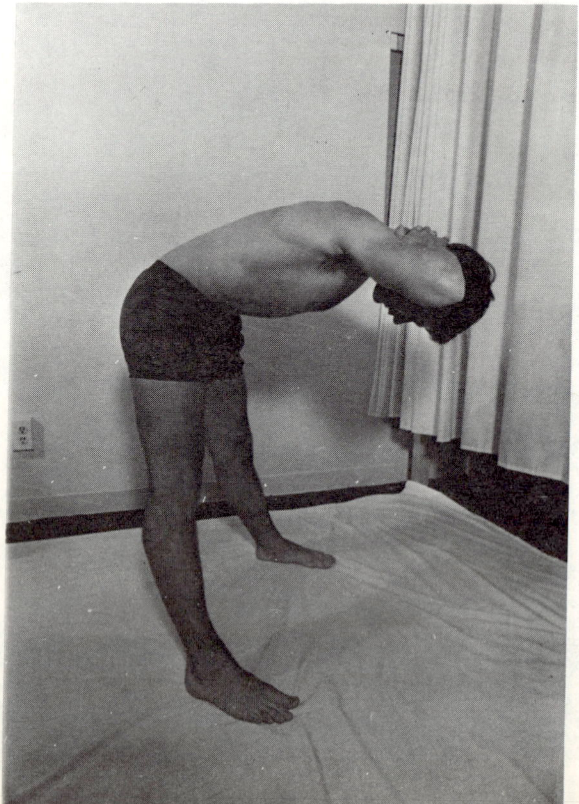

7

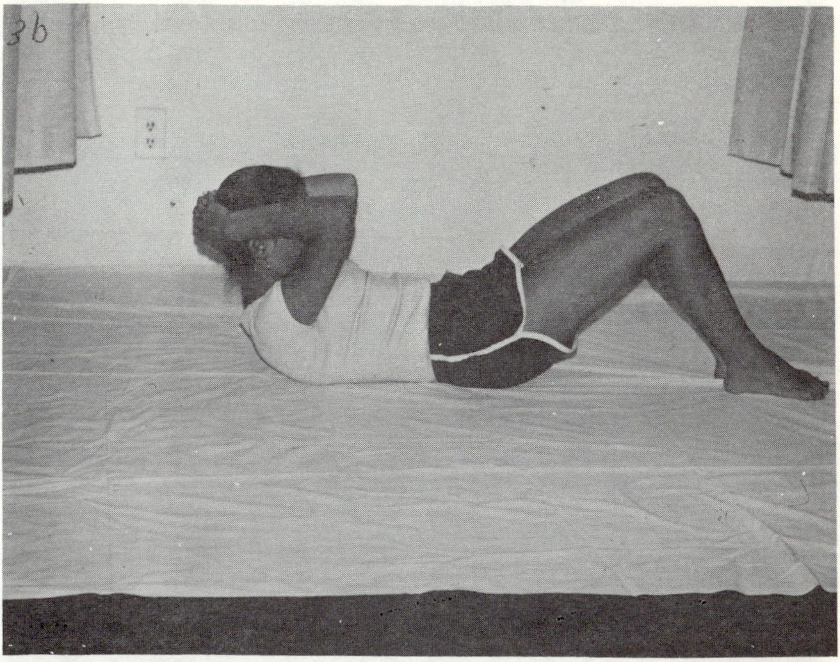

8

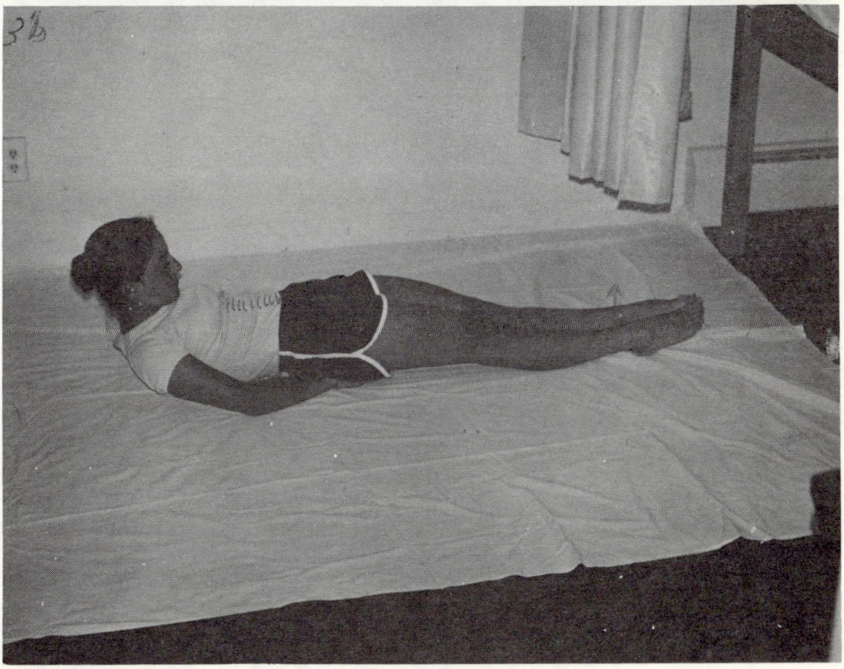

9

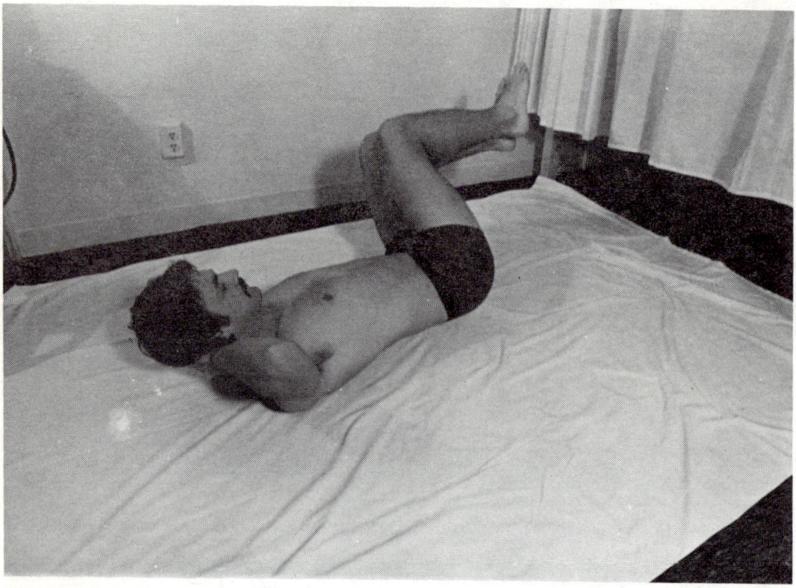

10

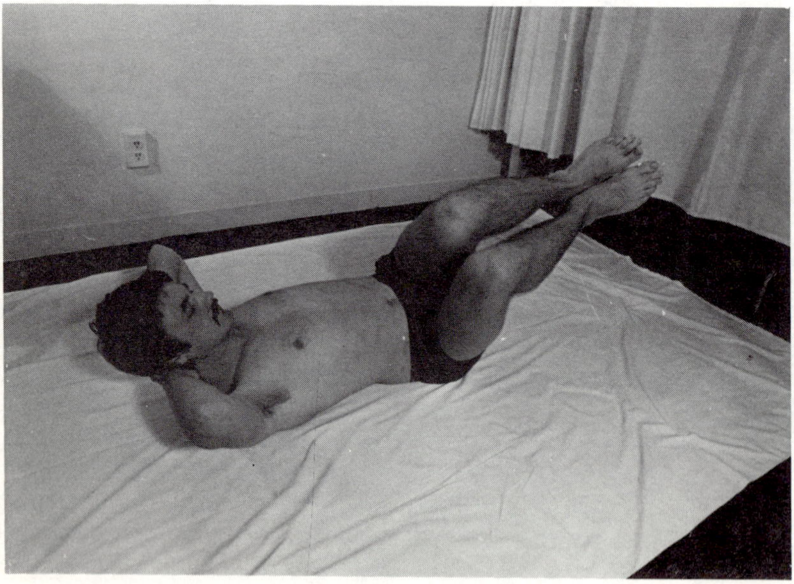

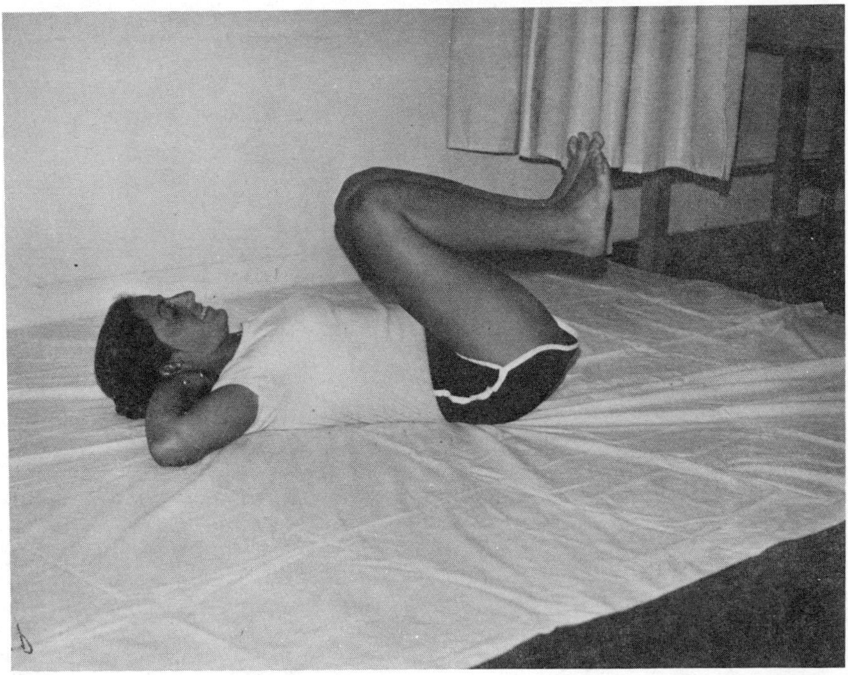

11a

11b

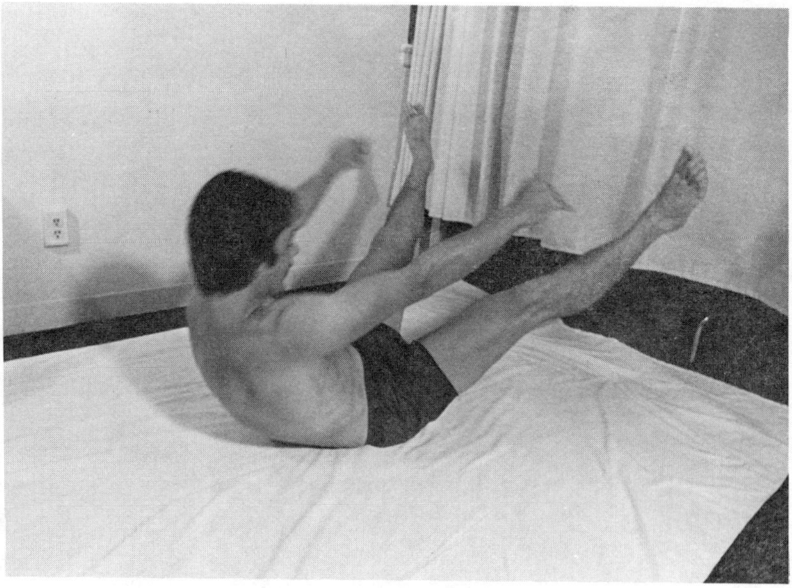

12a

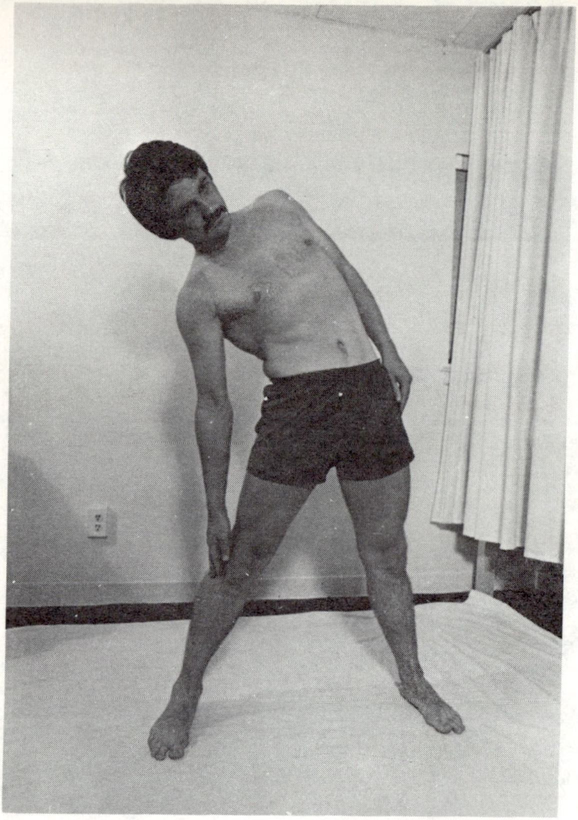

12b

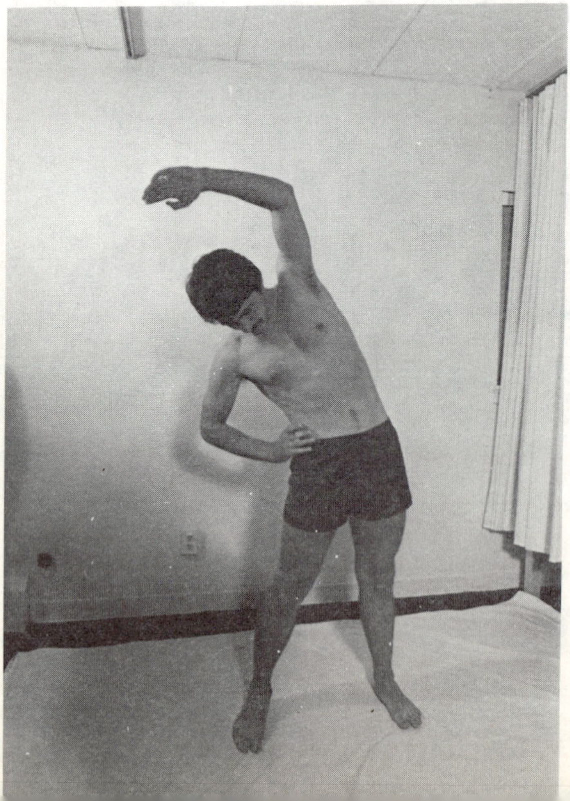

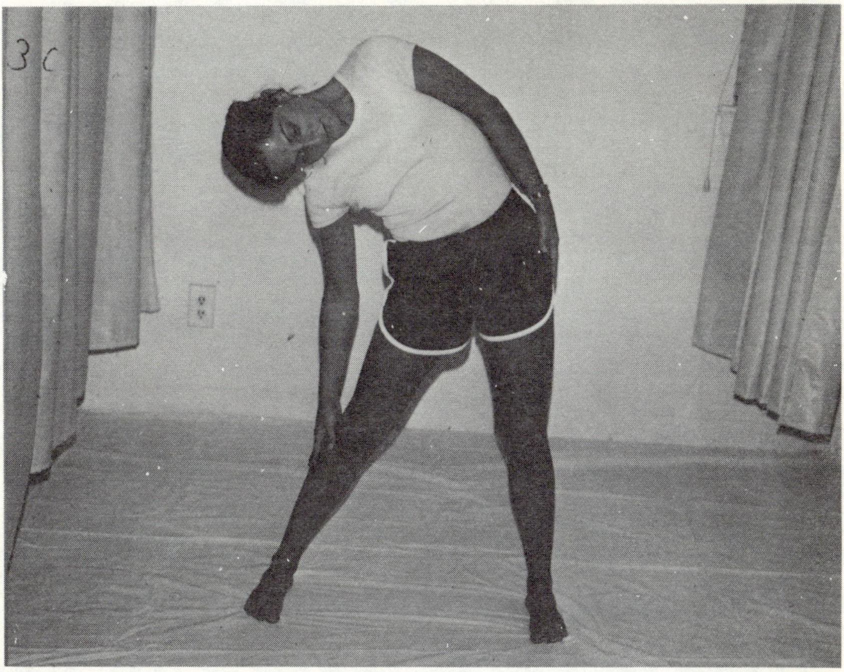

12c

9. Stengthening lower abdominals and obliques.

10. Strengthening lower hip muscles (anteriorly) and obliques.

11a, b. Strengthening abdominal, lower abdominal, and hip flexors.

12. Stretching lateral muscles of the body and trunk in three different positions, a, b, c.

Figure 80B. Lateral and Medial Muscles of the Body

13. Strengthening abductors (gluteus medius).

14. Strengthening abductors (tenso-fasciae latae)—this muscle abducts thigh when it is placed 30-40 degrees in forward hip flexion.

15. Strengthening adductors (inside the thigh).

16. Strengthening hip abductors (left leg forward and upward).

17. Strengthening right medial muscles (adductors).

18. Same as position #16 except greater flexibility by female athletes.

13 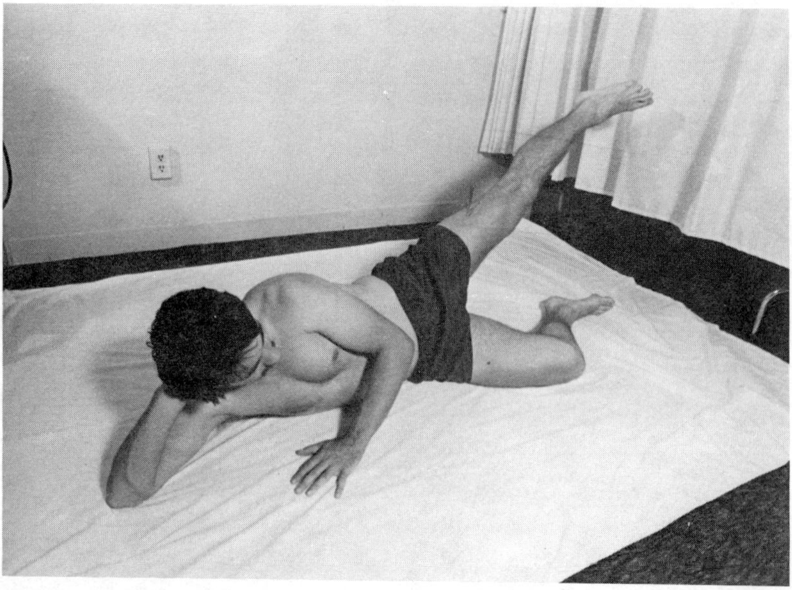

Figure 80b. Stretching and strenthening the Lateral and Medial muscles of the body.

14 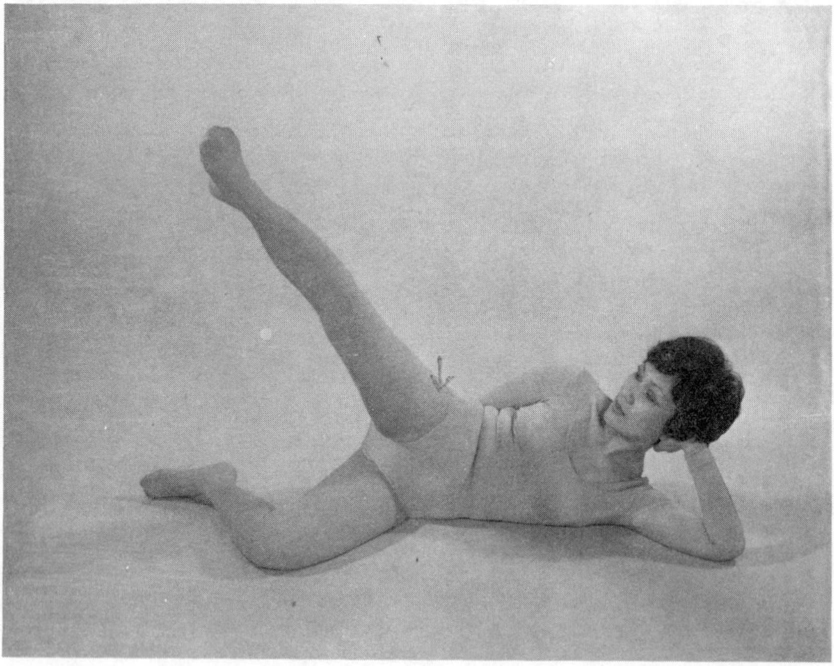

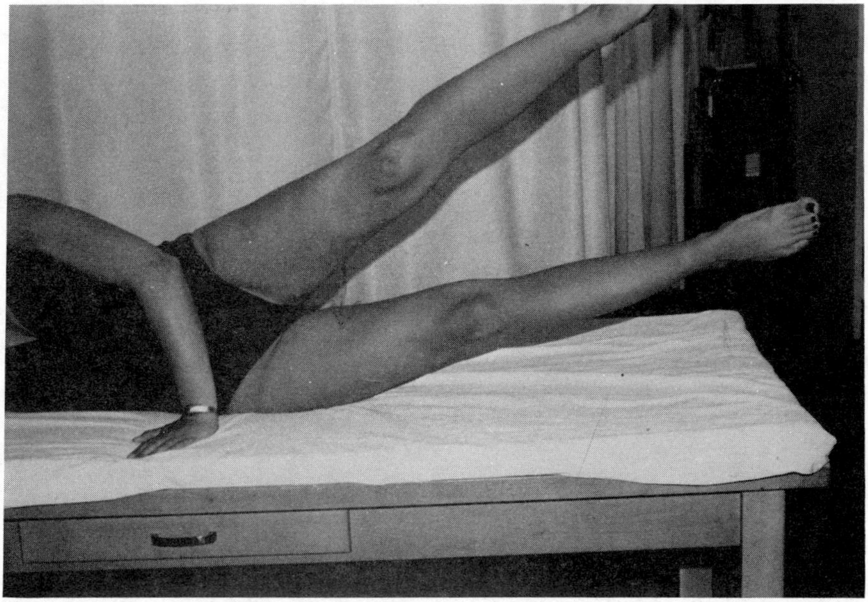

15

16

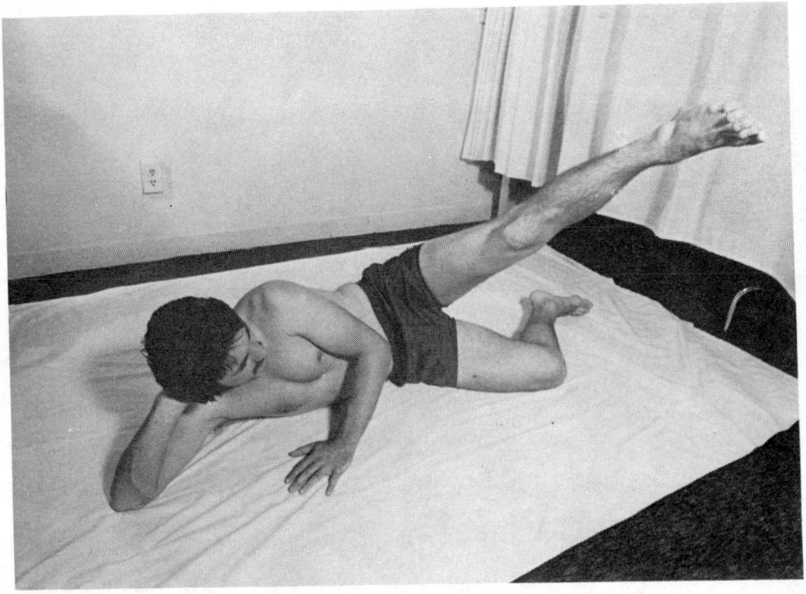

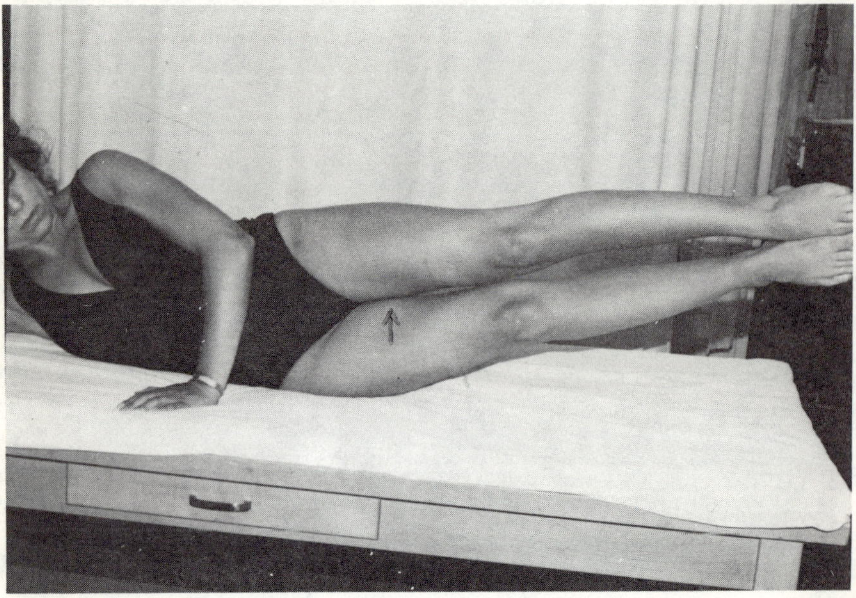

17

18

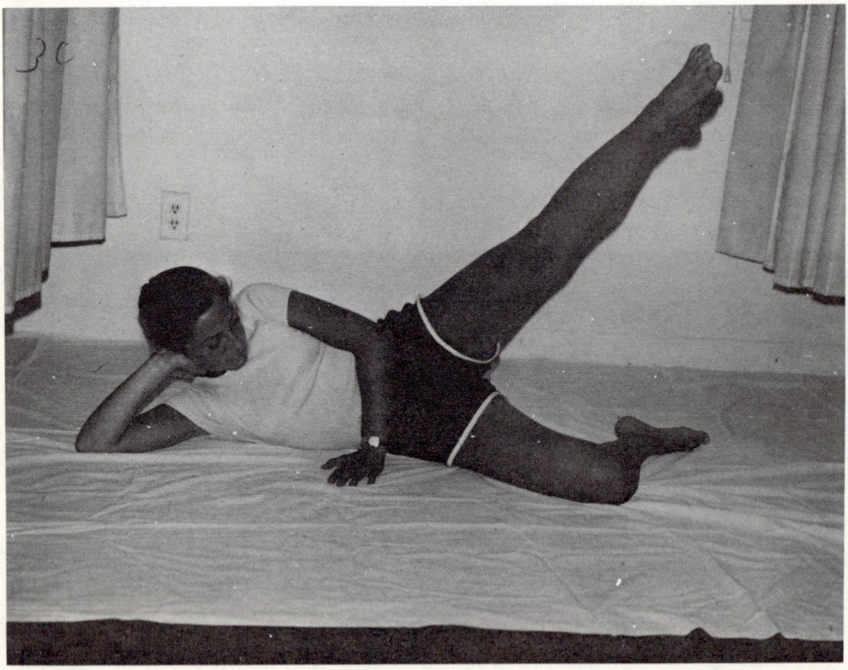

Figure 81. Strengthening the posterior (back) muscles of the upper and lower back against gravity and against resistance.

1. Thoracic and lumbar spine.
2. Gluteus and hamstrings (hips and thighs).
3. Stretching upper and lower spine.
4. Strengthening upper and lower spine musculature.
5. Strengthening upper spine and shoulder proper.
6. Gluteus maximus only, with knees flexed to 90 degrees (hips only).
7. P.R.E. strengthening gluteus with weights placed at the ankle and leg, providing a resistive force (see arrow 1). Arrow 2 represents the site of the contraction.
8. Strengthening gluteus assisted with weights by hamstring.
9. Strengthening posterior (back) muscles (spine, shoulder blade, and hip musculature).
10. Strengthening upper thoracic spine and cervical extensors.
11. Strengthening gluteus and lumbar musculature (hips and lower back).
12. Coordination exercise of upper and lower posterior muscles of spine, hips, and shoulder. (multifidus)

1

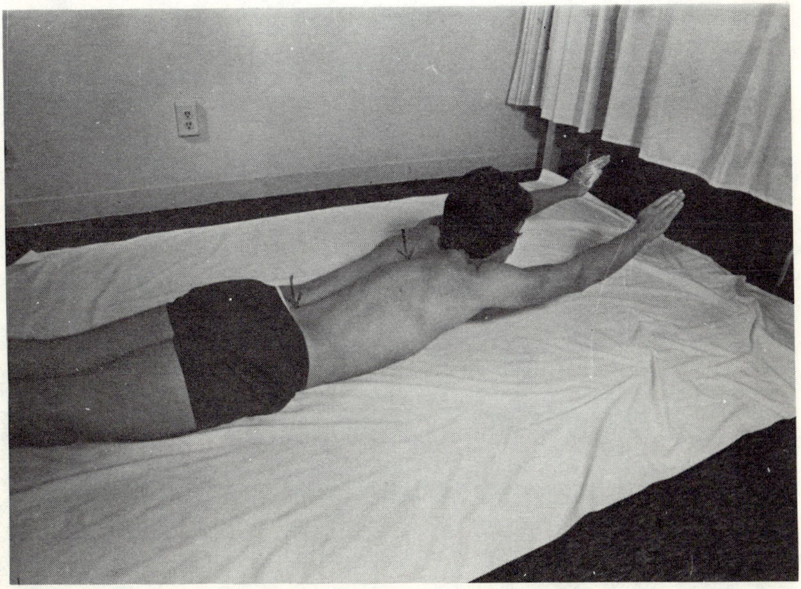

Figure 81. Strengthening the Posterior (Back) muscles of the upper and lower back.

Fig. 81

2

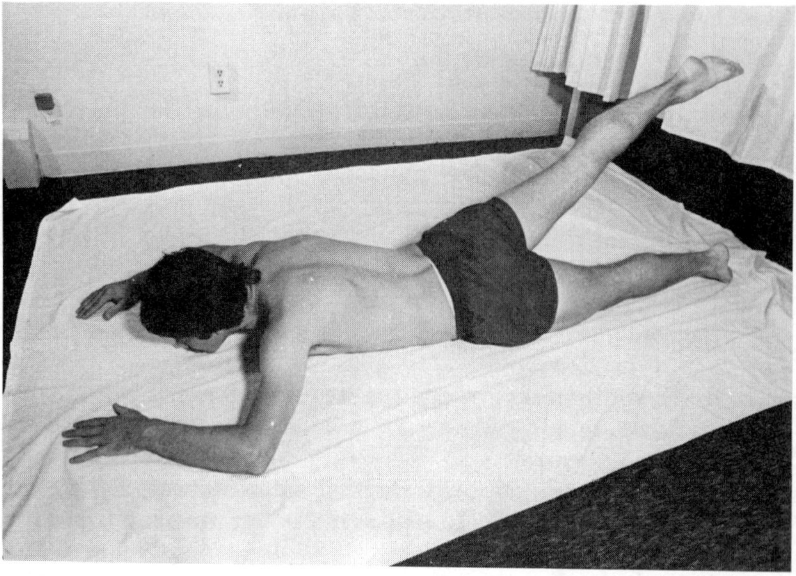

3

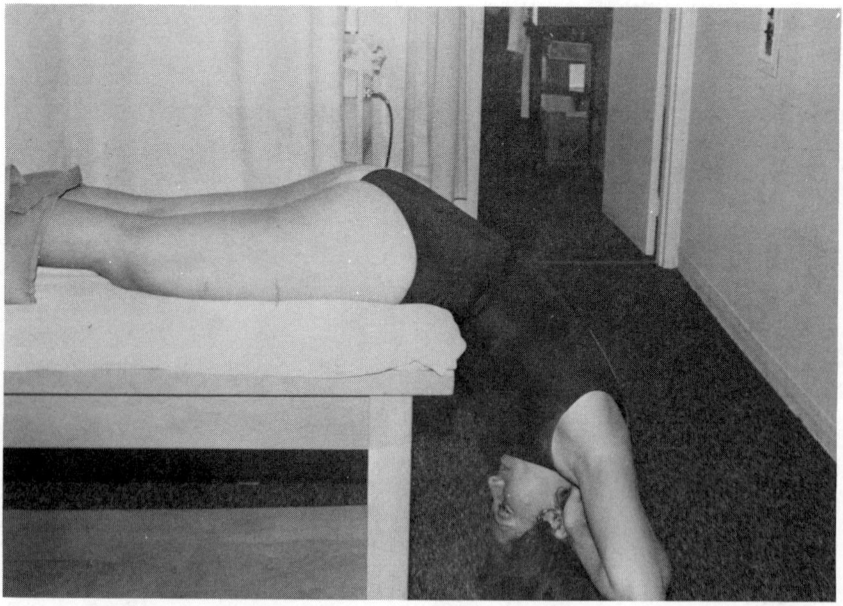

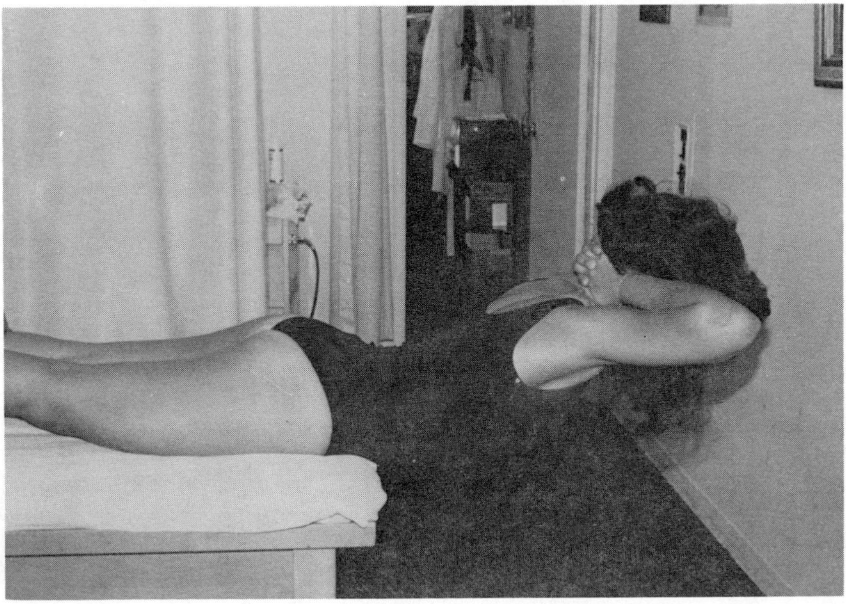

4

5

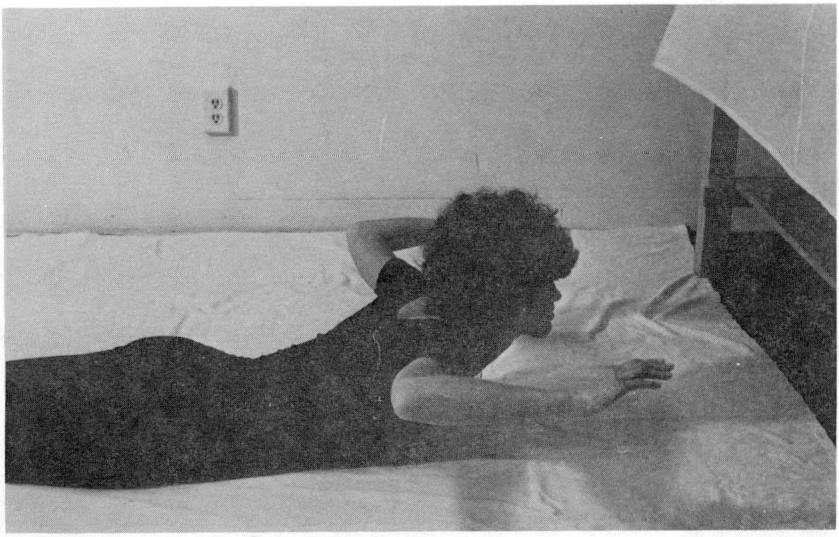

Fig. 81 Continued

6

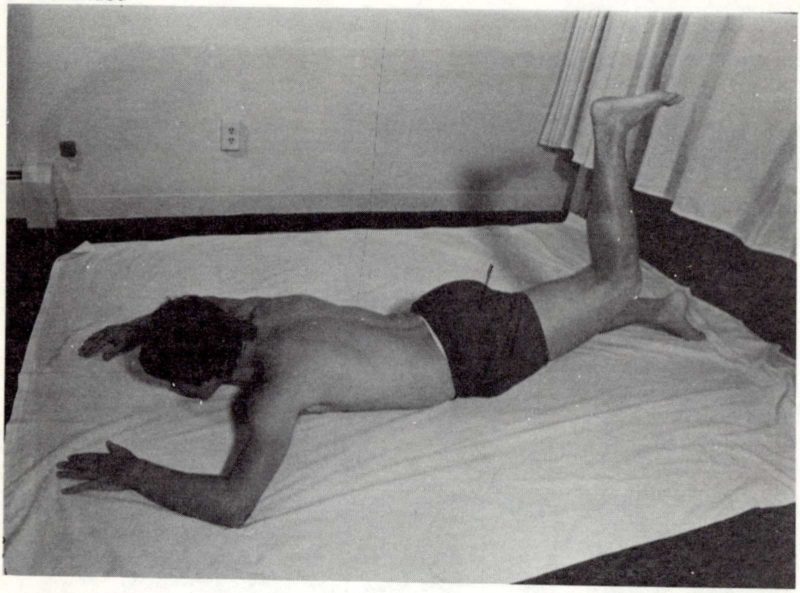

7

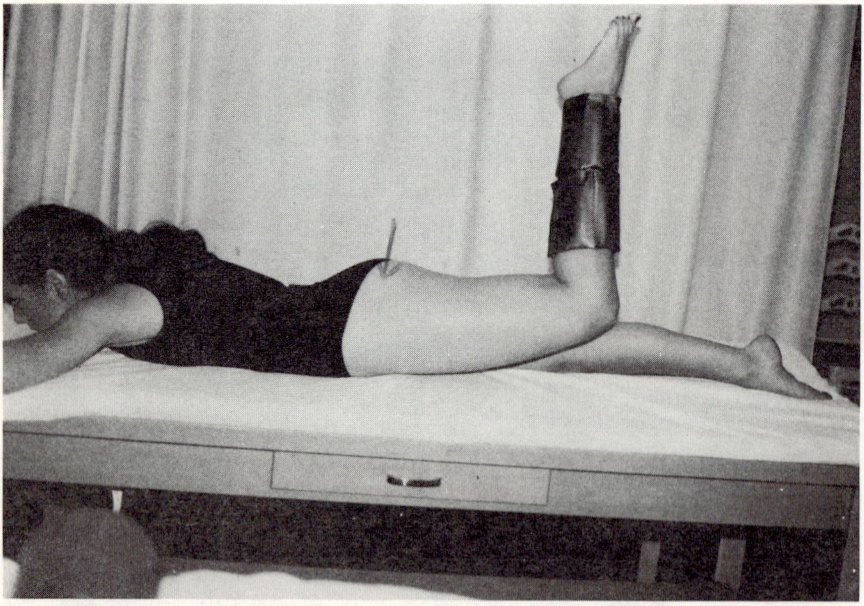

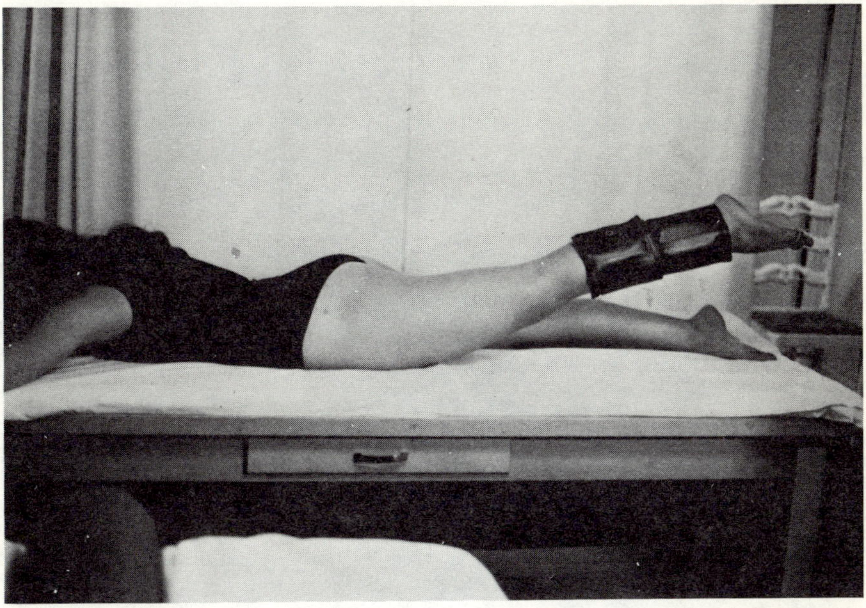

8

9

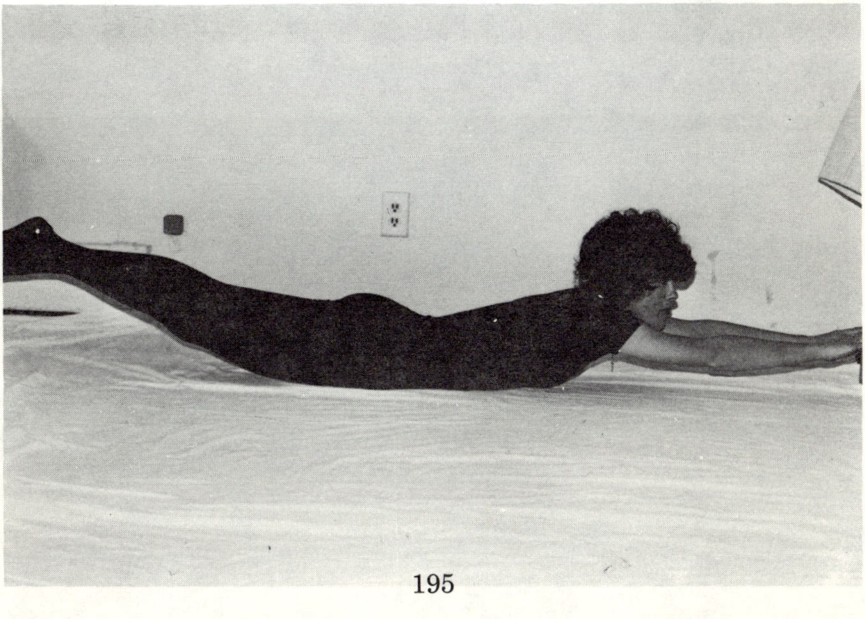

Fig. 81 Continued

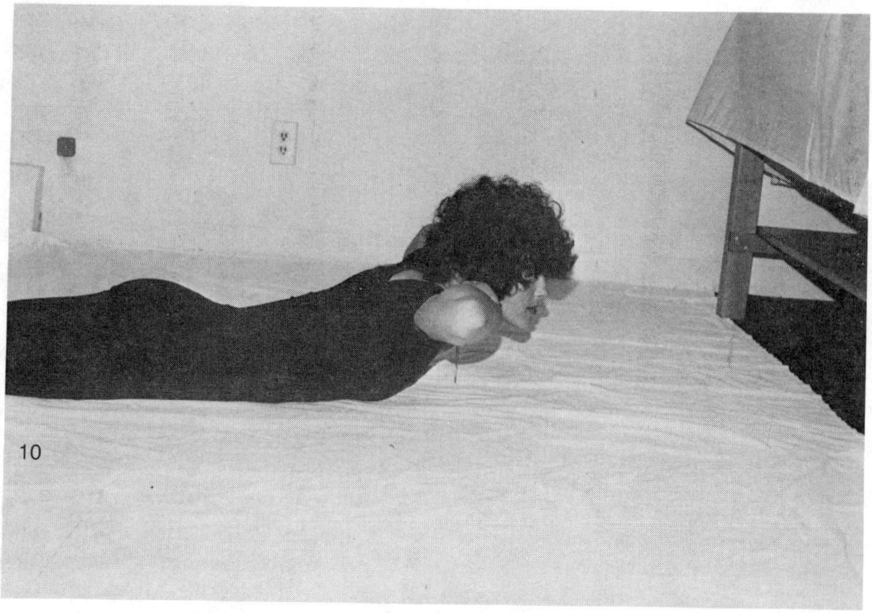

10

11

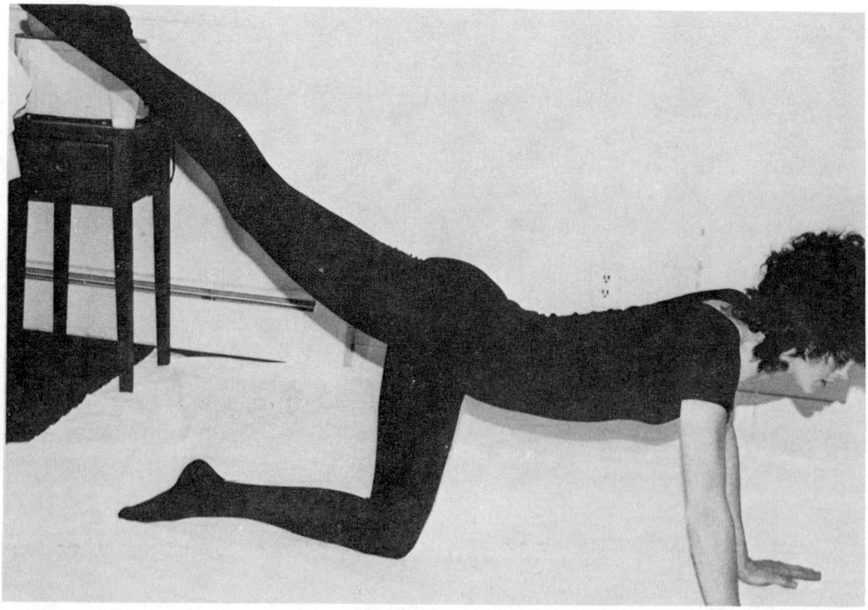

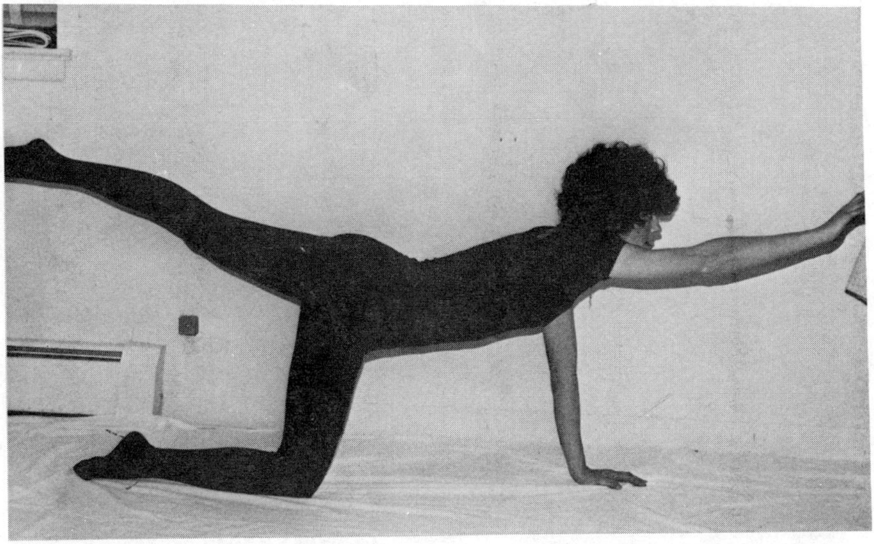

12

Figure 82. Stretching the anterior (front) muscles (hip flexors and knee extensors) in the prone and supine positions and strengthening the hip extensors without weights.

1. Stretching knee extensors (quadriceps) actively.
2. Self-applied stretching of hip flexors and knee extensors.
3. Self-applied stretching bilaterally of knee extensors (quadriceps).
4. Stretching the hip extensors (glutei) and hip flexors simultaneously.
5. Stretching the hip extensors in prone position. (Note: The pelvis must remain down (see arrow).
6. Strengthening hip extensors with the assistance of the hamstrings.

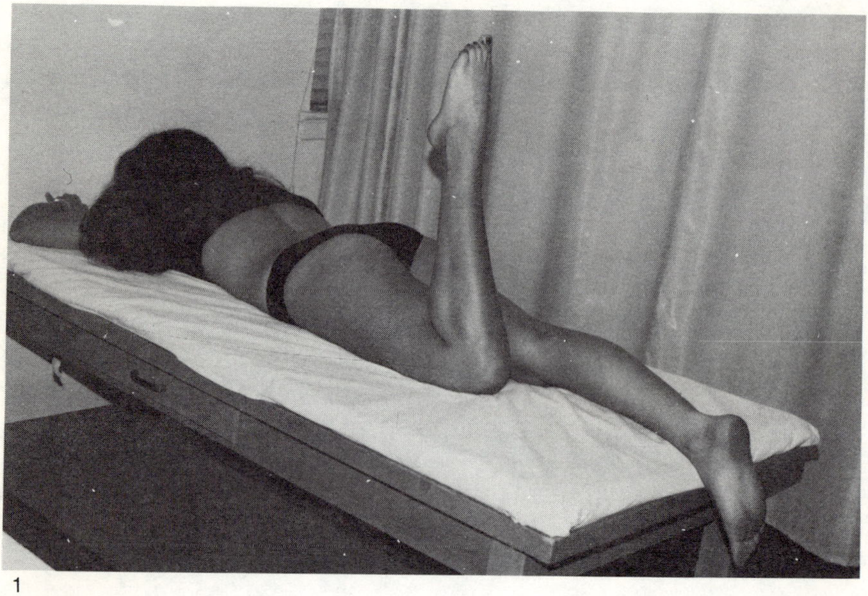

1

Figure 82. Stretching the Anterior (Front) muscles (Hip flexors and knee extensors) in the prone and supine positions, and strengthening the hip extensors without weights.

2

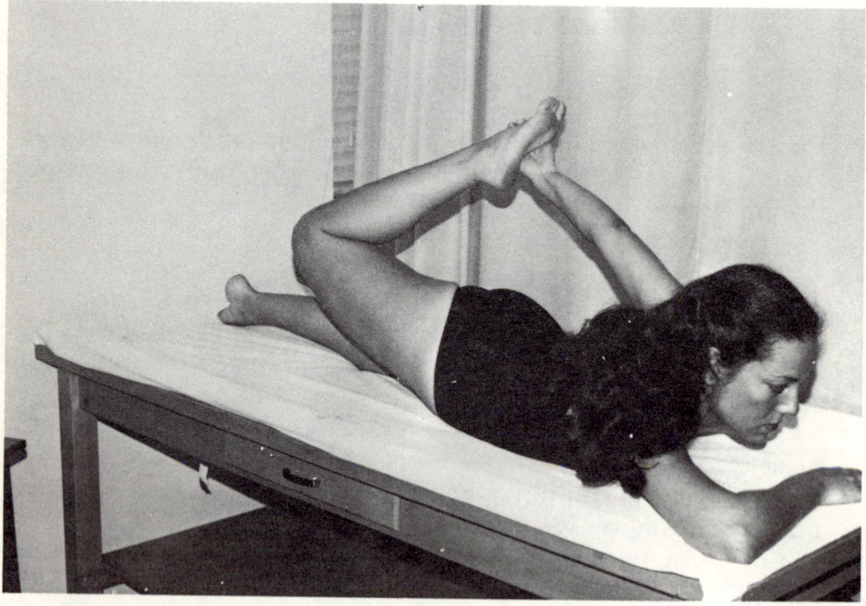

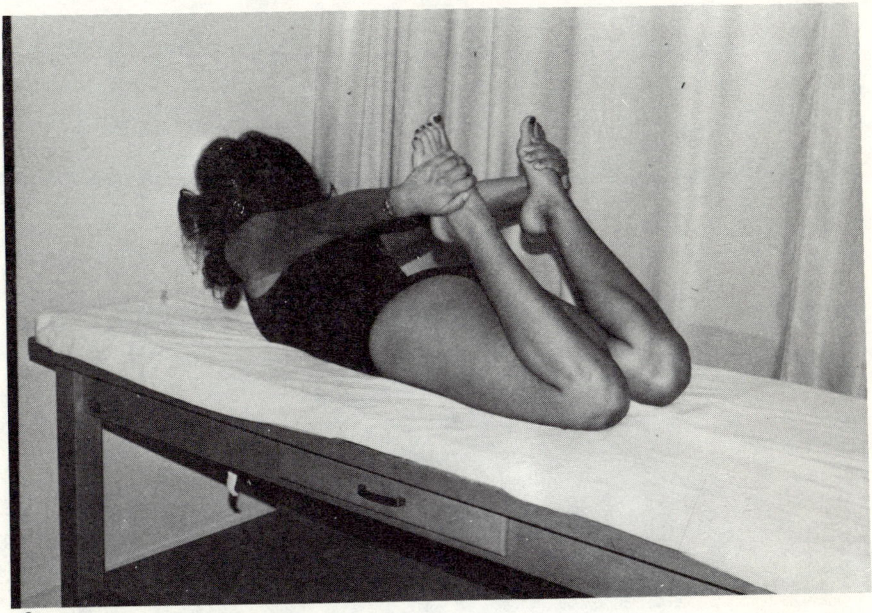

3

4

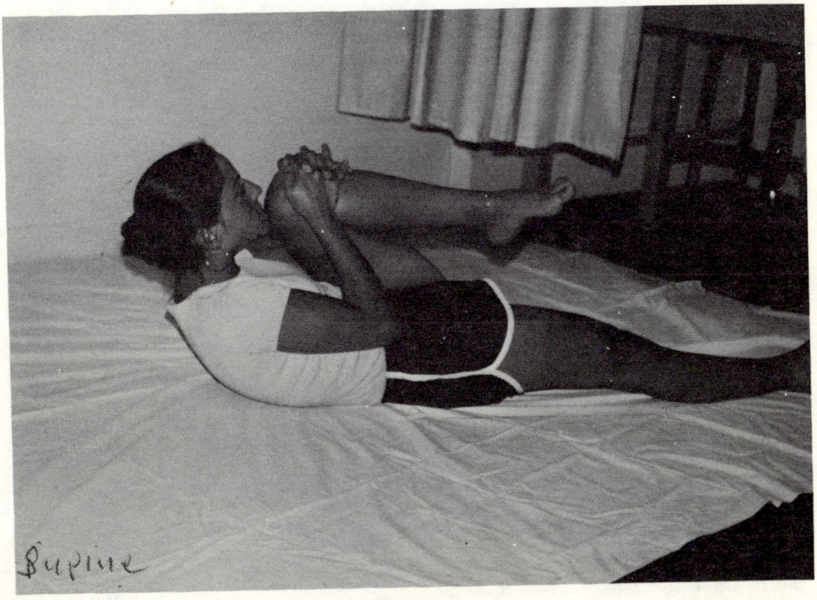

Fig. 82 Continued

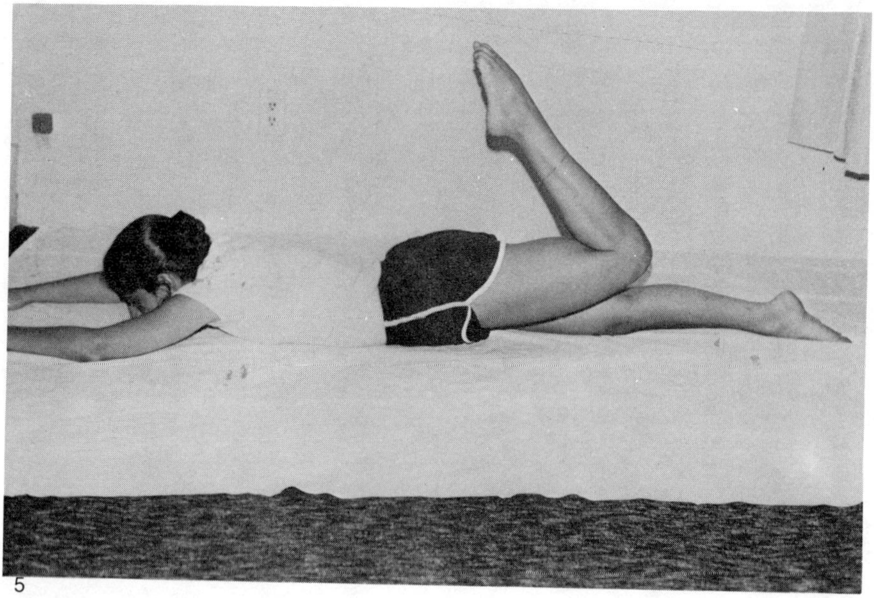

5

6

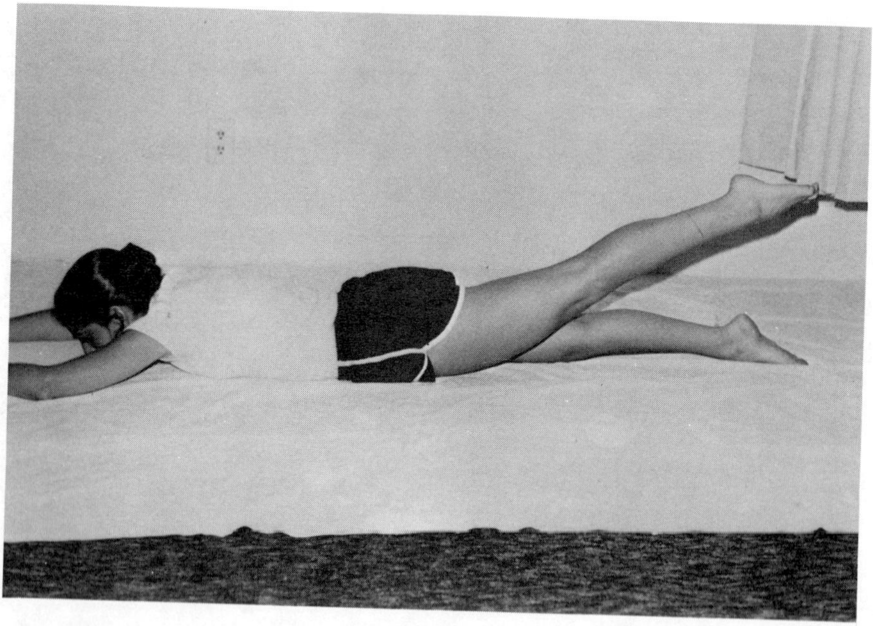

Figure 83. Strengthening the muscles of the arm and shoulder.

1. Four points of support: hands and knees, for beginners.
2. Four points of support: hands and dorsal or volar part of feet and toes, for more advanced.
3. Completion of pushup: chest and chin are touching the floor.

1

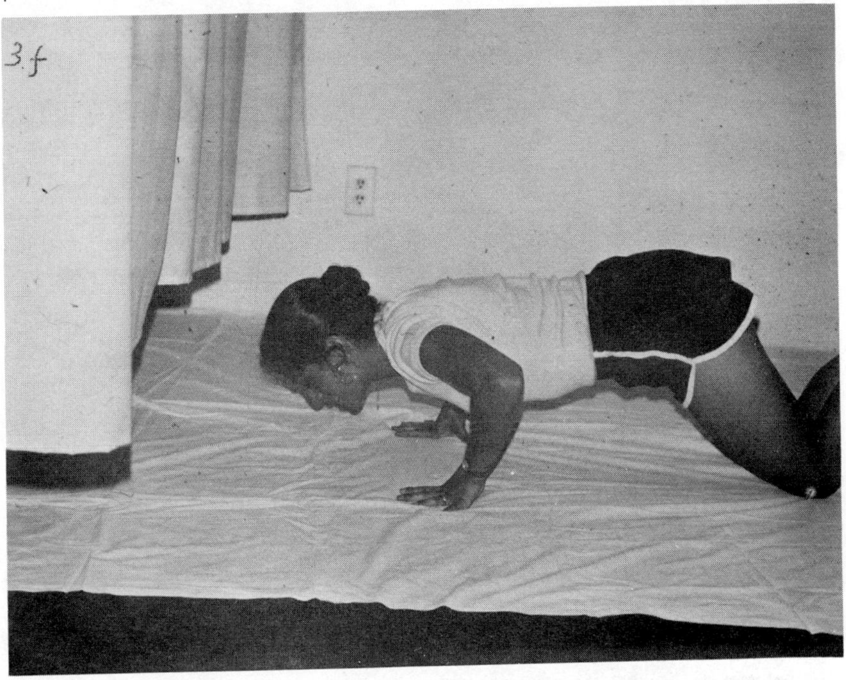

Figure 83. Strengthening the muscles of the arm and shoulder (Normal pushup for beginners and more advanced).

Fig. 83 Continued

2

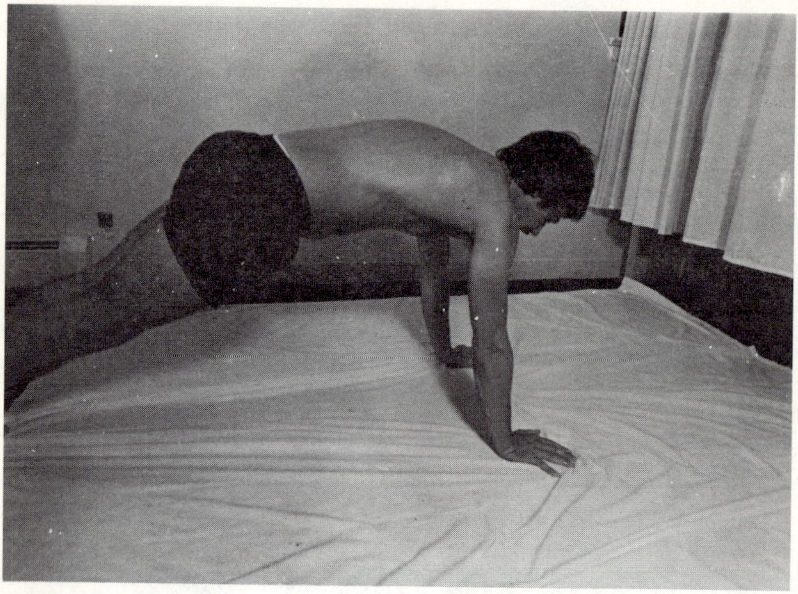

3

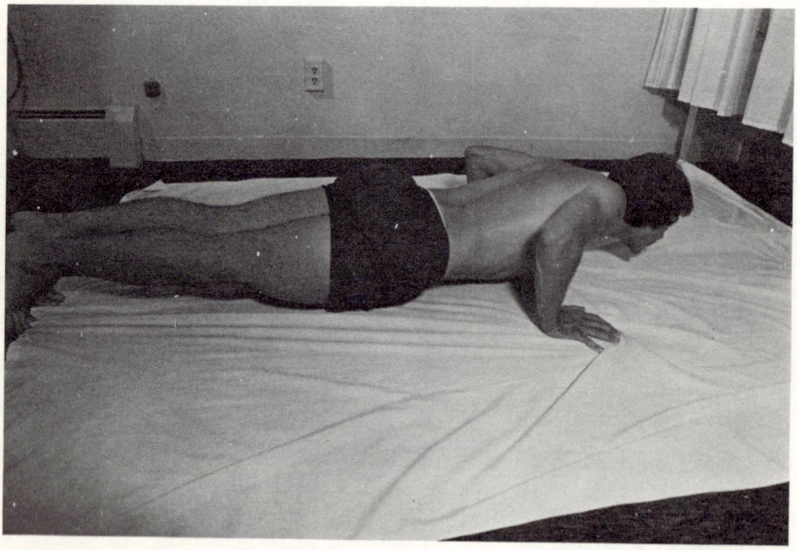

Figure 84. Advanced push-ups (4 stages).

All four stages contribute in stretching and strengthening the anterior and posterior muscles of the body while their prime action is concentrated in strengthening muscles of the shoulder and arms. This type of push-up is a very advanced one.

1

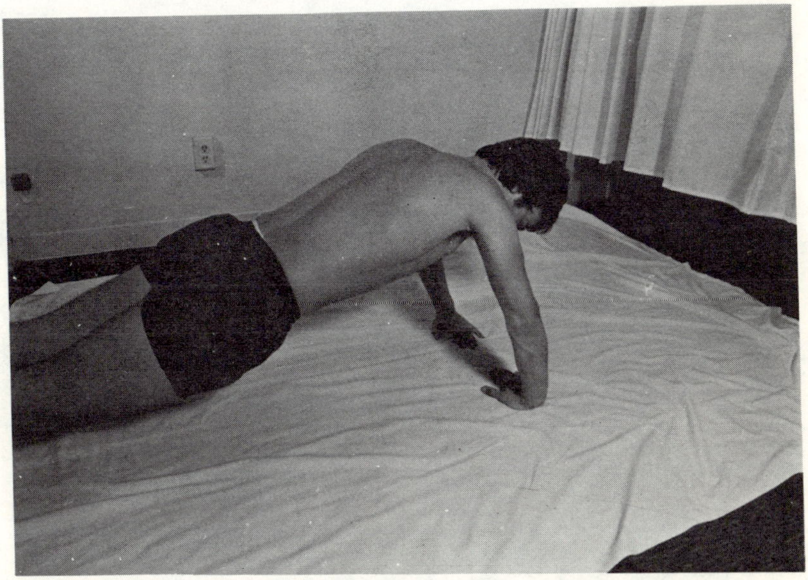

Figure 84. Four stages of the Pushup (Arching the spine at the same time).

Fig. 84 continued

2

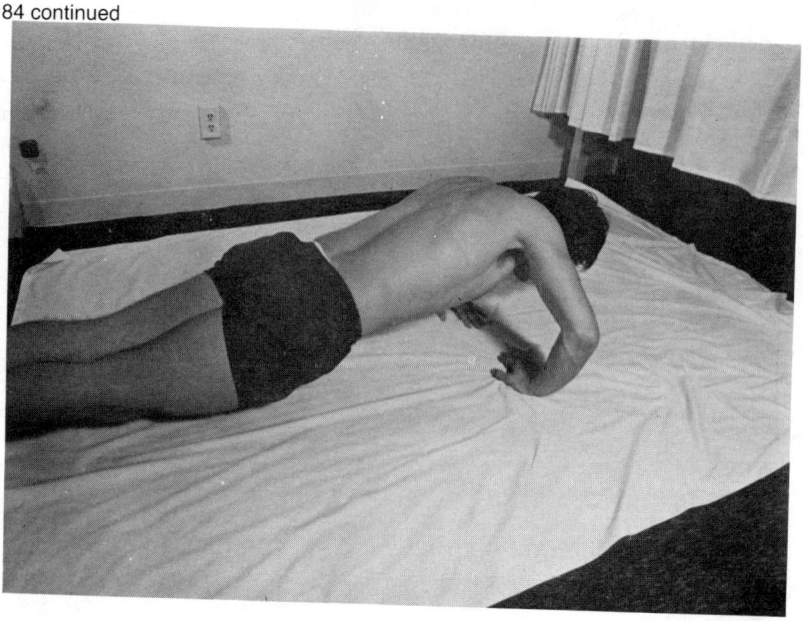

3

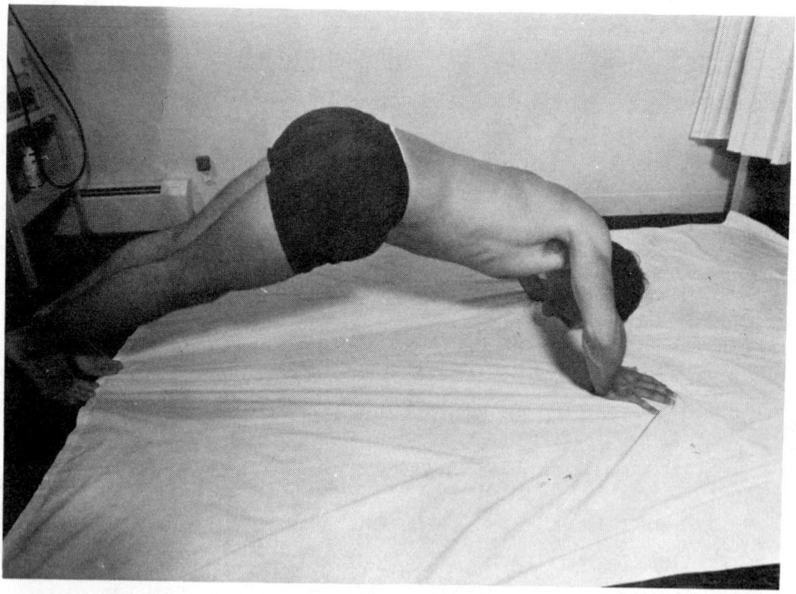

4 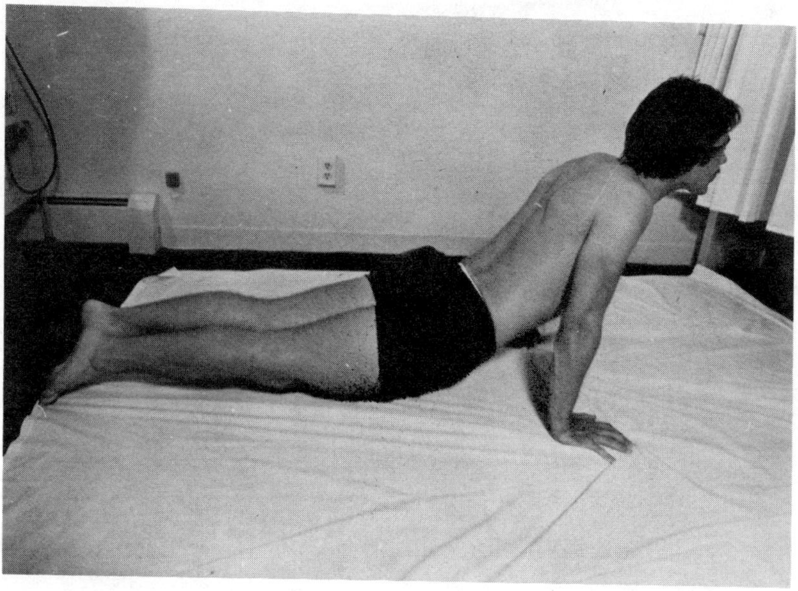

Figure 85. Trunk, lateral flexion and rotation for maximum exertion to increase the vital pathways of the respiratory system.

1. Trunk, lateral flexion: right hand assisting sideward thrust of the trunk.
2. Lateral flexion with hands behind neck and chest out.
3. Trunk rotation with arms abducted (at shoulder level) to increase the force of rotation.
4. Combination of trunk rotation and extension.
5. Combination of trunk rotation and flexion.

1

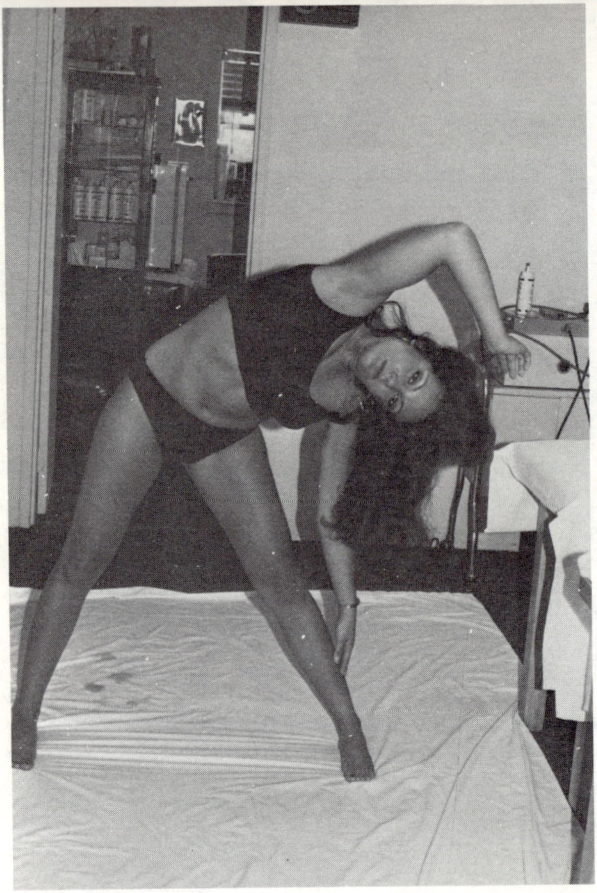

Figure 85. Trunk, Lateral flexion, and rotation for maximum exertion to increase the vital pathways of the respiratory system.

2

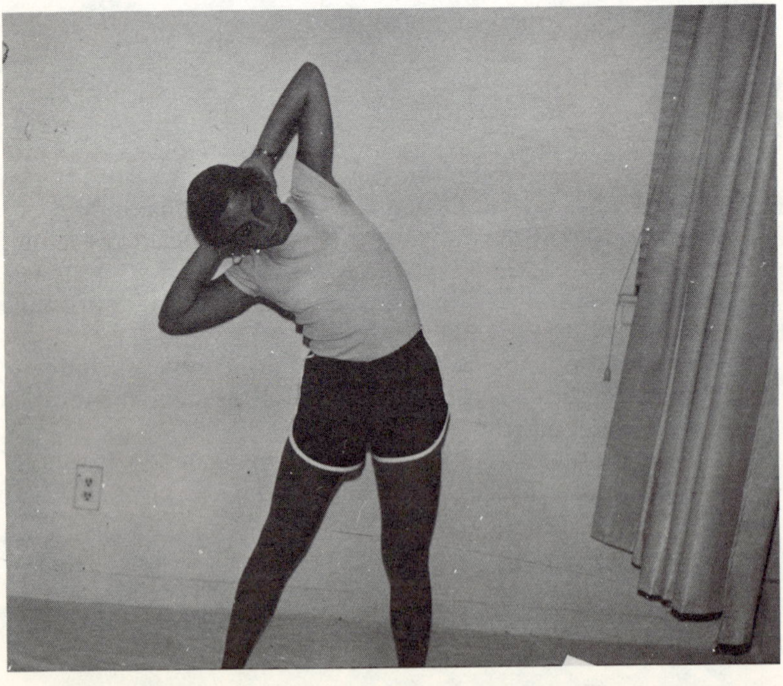

3

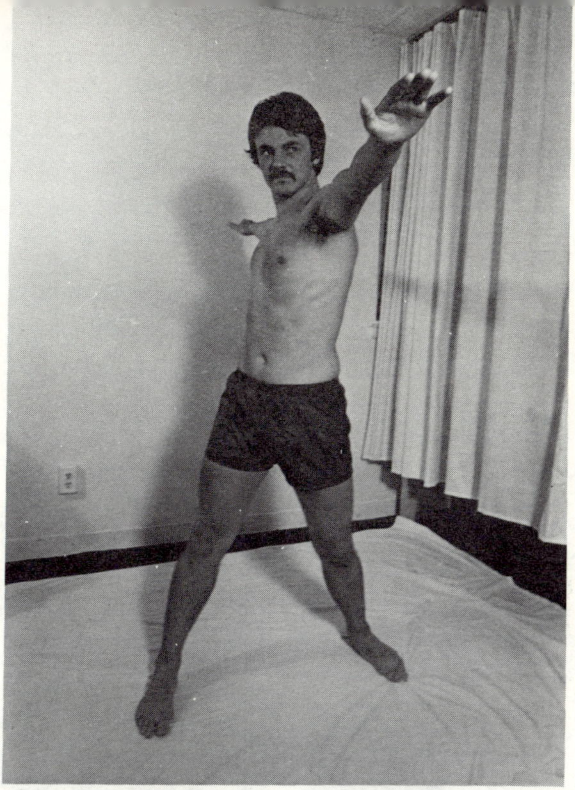

4

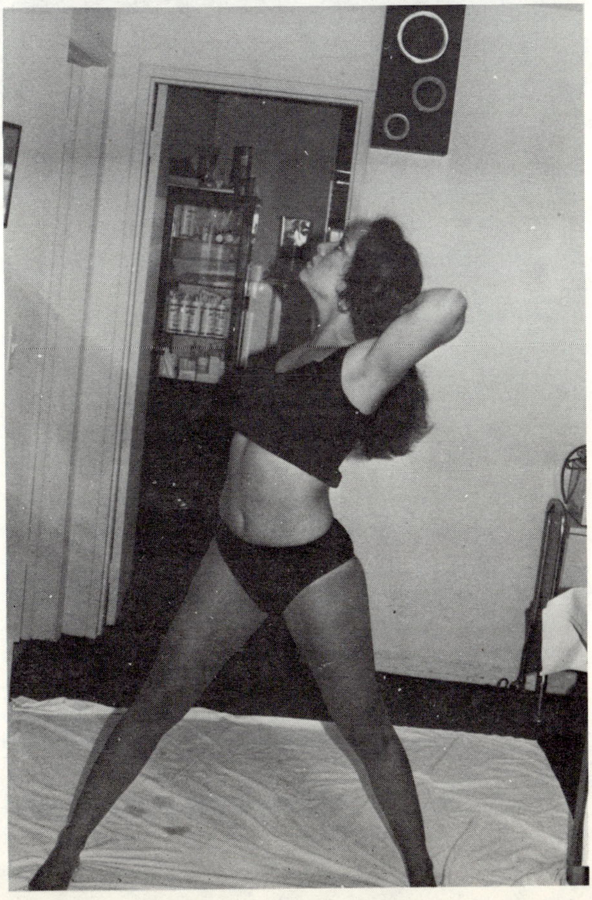

Fig. 86 continued

5

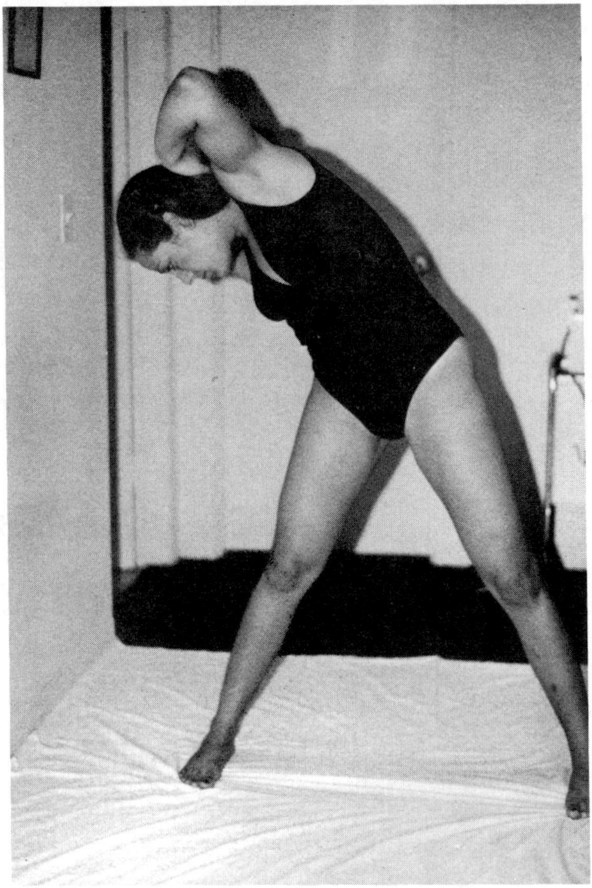

Figure 86. Neck, lateral flexion and rotation as well as forward flexion and extension.

1. Lateral flexion to the right with arms abducted (right ear touching right shoulder).
2. Lateral flexion to the right with hands on hips.
3. Neck rotation with arms extended to shoulder level.
4. Neck rotation with hands on hips.
5. Neck extension.
6. Neck forward flexion (chin touches chest).

Note: All stretching exercises should be performed very slowly. Any sudden movement may result in muscle pulls. During muscle stretching and/or strengthening, once the desired position has been completed, it should be maintained in this position for at least 6 seconds or a slow count from 1 to 6. These exercises are vital for the player's health, physical fitness, and the best prevention of injuries. However, when injury does occur, these exercises, when performed in the aforementioned progression, provide the means for total rehabilitation.

1

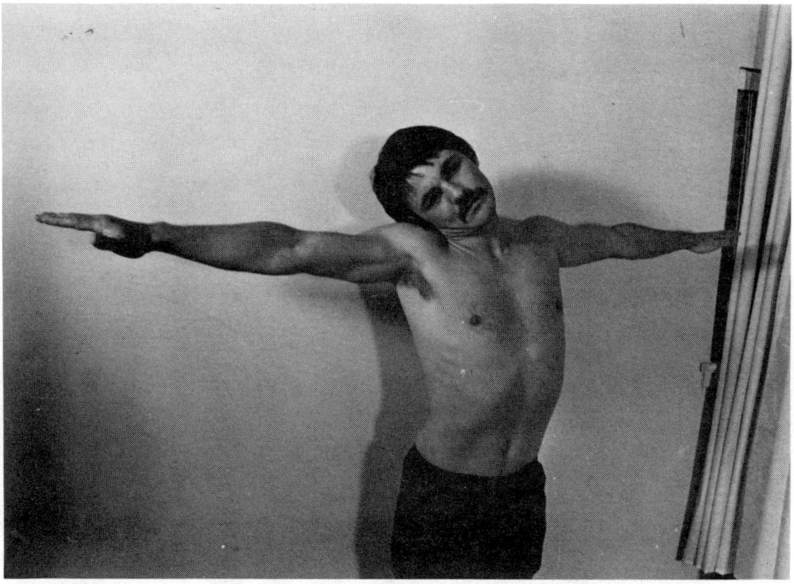

Figure 86. Neck, Lateral flexion and rotation as well as forward flexion and extension.

Fig 86 continued

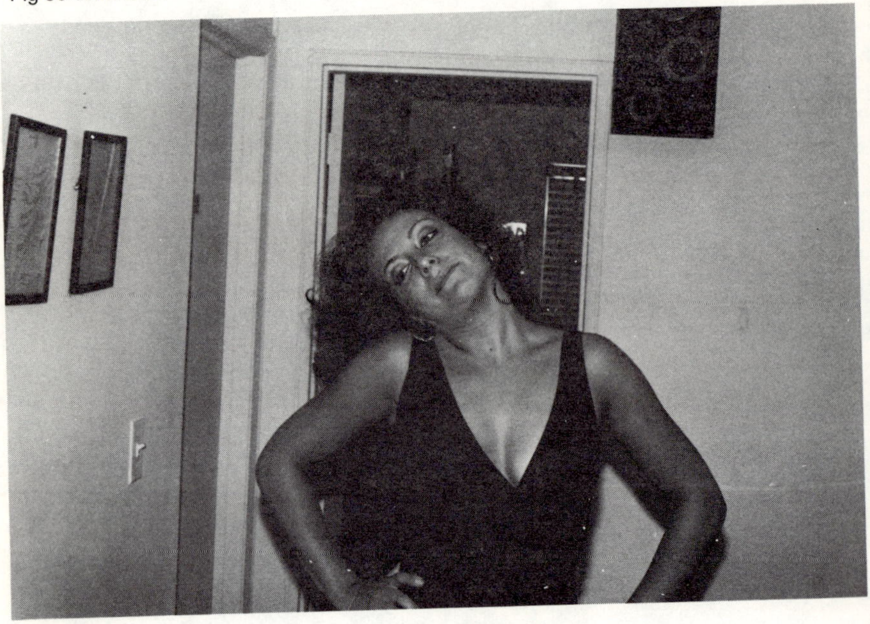

2

3

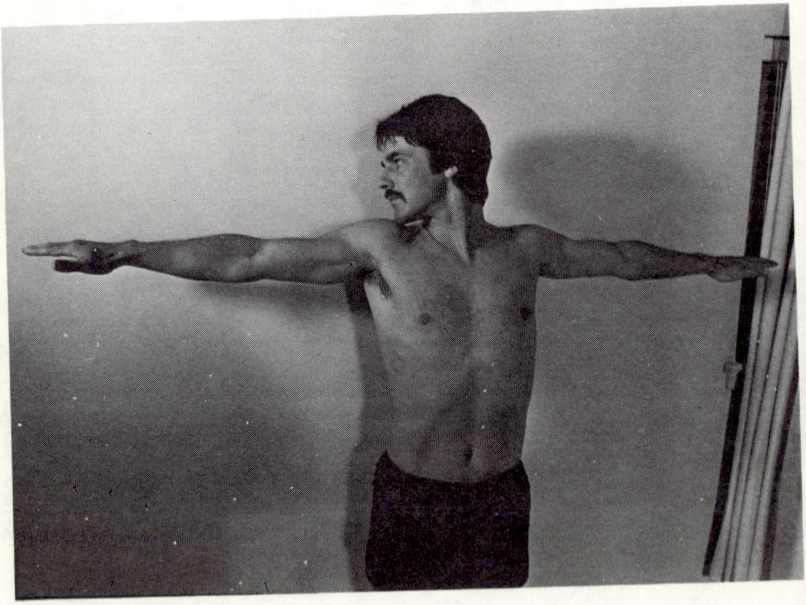

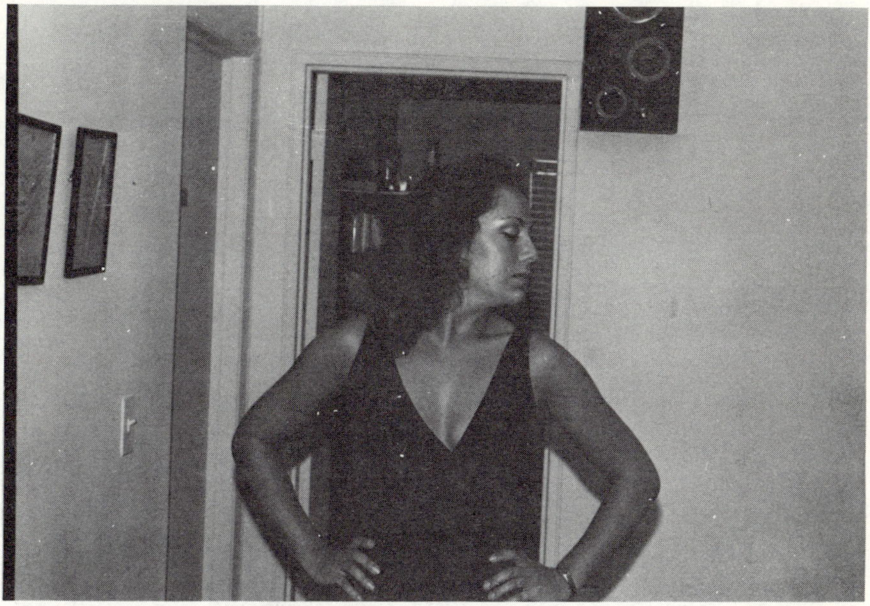

4

5

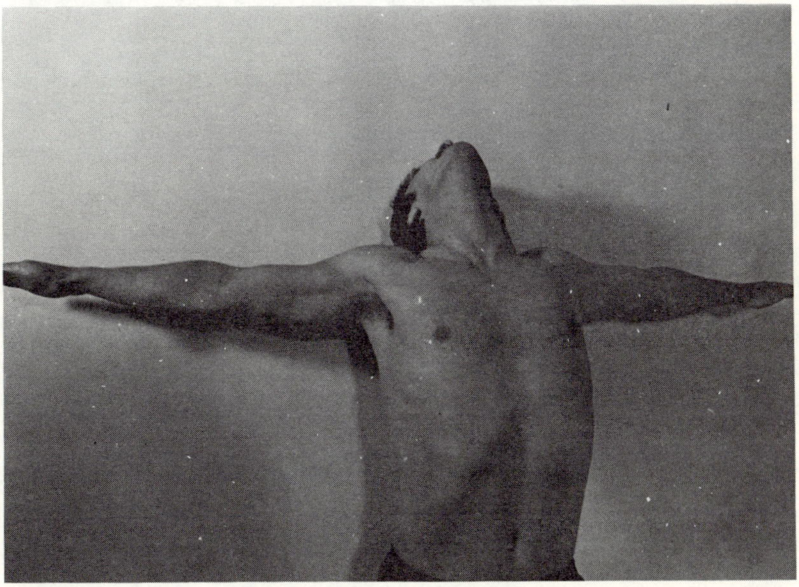

Fig 86 continued

6 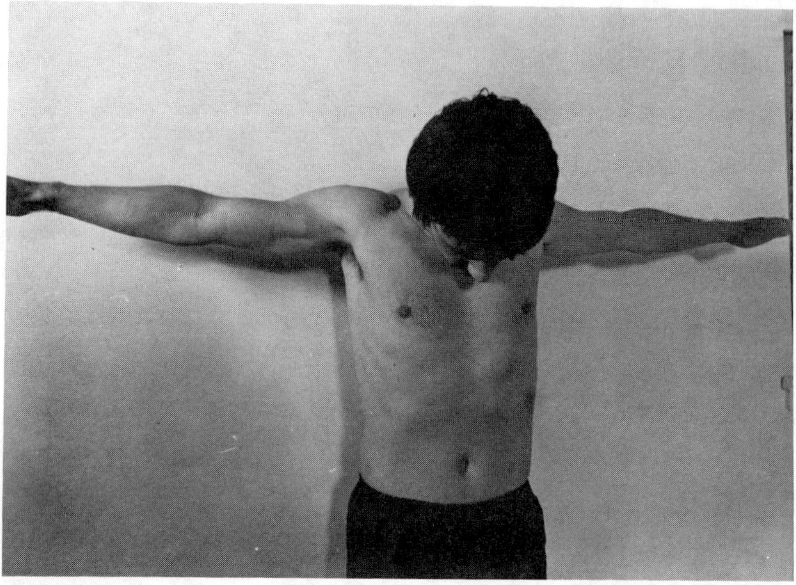

Bibliography

1. Avgerinos, Nicholas. "Physicotherapeia: Most Recent Approach in Treating Traumatic Shoulder," *Pan Hellenic Physiotherapy Society Journal*, Volume 2, (September 1979).
2. Bailey, Robert W. "Myology, Cervical Spine Disorders: Diagnosis and Treatment," *A.H. Robins Monographs for Continuing Education*, Volume 1, Number 2, (Summer 1976).
3. Best, Charles Herbert and Payala, Norman Burke *The Living Body, A Text in Human Physiology*. London and Canada: Henry Holt and Company, 1952.
4. Bloomberg, Maxwell H. *Orthopedic Braces: Rationale, Classification, and Prescription,* Philadelphia: J.P. Lippincott Co., 1964.
5. Blyth, Carl S. and Mueller, Frederick, O. "Football Injuries," *Physicians and Sports Medicine,* McGraw-Hill, Inc., 1974.
6. Bugaj, Ronald. "The Cooling Analgesic," *Journal of the A.P.T.A.*, Volume 55, (January 1975).
7. Cailliet, Rene. *Neck and Arm Pain*. Philadelphia: F.A. Davis, 1972.
8. Cerney, J.V. *An Encyclopedia of Causes, Effects and Treatment of Athletes,* Springfield, Ill.: Charles C. Thomas, 1963.
9. Cramer, Dettmar. *Coach's Manual*. Minisink Hill, Penn: Four Maples Press, 1973.
10. Daniels, Lucille, and Williams, Marian, and Worthingham, Catherine. *Muscle Testing, Techniques of Manual Examination*. Philadelphia: W.B. Saunders Co., 1961.
11. Dayton, O. William. *Athletic Training and Conditioning*. New York: Ronald Press, 1960.
12. Demarest, Robert J. *Medical Illustrations of Common Traumatic Conditions*. Indianapolis, Indiana; Eli Lilly and Co., Nov., 1969.
13. Ducroquet, Robert, and Ducroquet, Jean, and Ducroquet, Pierre. *Walking and Limping: A Study of Normal and Pathological Walking*. Philadelphia: J.B. Lippincott Co., 1968.
14. Etheredge, Maude Lee. *Health Facts for College Students*. Philadelphia: W.B. Saunders and Co., 1953.
15. Fralick, Samuel. *Soccer*. New York: A.S. Barnes and Co., 1945.
16. Gardner, Ernest, Gray, D.J., and O'Rahilly, R. *Anatomy: A Regional Study of Human Structure*. Phildelphia: W.B. Saunders Co., 1960.
17. Goodgold, Joseph. *Anatomical Correlates of Clinical Electromyography*. Baltimore: Williams and Wilkins Co., 1974.
18. Gray, Henry and Gross, Mayo. *Gray's Anatomy* (28th Edition), Philadelphia: Lea and Febiger, 1968.
19. Hollinshead, W. Henry. *Functional Anatomy of the Limbs and Back*. Philadelphia: W.B. Saunders and Co., 1960.

20. Hosking, M.R. *Bandaging Made Easy*. London: Faber and Faber, LTD, 1945.
21. Jokl, Ernst, and Simon, E. *International Research in Sports and Physical Education*. Springfield, Ill.: Charles C. Thomas, 1964.
22. Krusen, and Kottke, and Ellwood, *Handbook of Physical Medicine and Rehabilitation*. Philadelphia: W.B. Saunders Co., 1968.
23. Lammich, Gunther and Kadow, Heinz. *Warm-up For Soccer*. New York: Sterling Publishing Co., 1975.
24. Leyshon, Glynn A. *Programmed Functional Anatomy*. St. Louis: C.V. Mosby Co., 1974.
25. Licht, Elizabeth and Licht, Sidney, ed., *Therapeutic Heat*. New Haven, Conn: 1958.
26. Lindquest, Jerome. *Approach to Electrotherapy*. Los Angeles, California: The Ward Ritchie Press, 1948.
27. Lurie, Jessie Zel and Seger, Samuel. *The Israel Army Physical Fitness*. New York: Grosset and Dunlap, 1969.
28. Menneli, John Mc M. *Joint Pain, Diagnosis, and Treatment Using Manipulative Techniques*. Boston: Little, Brown and Co., 1964.
29. Meyers, and Schwartz. *Team Sports for Girls and Women*. Philadelphia: W.B. Saunders Co., 1957.
30. Michele, Arthur. *Orthotherapy*. New York: M. Evans and Co., Inc., 1971.
31. Netter, Frank, H. *The Ciba Collection of Medical Illustrations*. Summit, N.J.: Ciba Pharmaceutical Products, Inc., 1953.
32. Novich, Max M. and Taylor, Buddy. *Training and Conditioning of Athletes*. Philadelphia: Lea and Febiger, 1970.
33. Ober, Frank R. *Backache*. Springfield, Ill.: Charles C. Thomas, 1955.
34. Pappan, Francis M. *Massage Techniques, A Case Method Approach*. New York: Macmillan Co., 1961.
35. Parry, C.W. Wynn. *Rehabilitation of the Hand*. London: Butterworth and Company, 1958.
36. Peebler, J.R. *Controlled Exercises for Physical Fitness*. Springfield, Ill: Charles C. Thomas, 1962.
37. Reed, J.D. SPORTS ILLUSTRATED (August 1977).
38. *Referees Charts and Players Guide to the Laws of Association Football*. Authorized by the International Football Association Board (Rev. Ed.) London and Sydney: Pan Books LTD, 1974.
39. Riedman, Sara R. *The Physiology of Work and Play*. Pennsylvania: Holt Driedman, Henry Holt and Co., 1974.
40. Rossman, Isadore, (ed.). *Clinical Geriatrics*., Philadelphia: Lippincott Co., 1971.
41. Scott, M. Gladys. *Analysis of Human Motion*. 2nd ed., New York: Appleton-Century Crofts, 1963.
42. Shands, Alfred Rieves. *Handbook of Orthopedic Surgery*. St. Louis: C.V. Mosby, 1957.
43. Thorndike, Jr., Augustus. *A Manual of Bandaging, Splinting, and Strapping*. Philadelphia: Lea and Febiger, 1941.
44. Wade, Allen. *Soccer, Guide to Training and Coaching*. New York: Funk and Wagnalls, 1967.
45. Walkins, Arthur L. *A Manual of Electrotherapy*. Philadelphia: Lea and Febiger, 1962.
46. Wolff, Harold G. and Wolf, Stewart. *Pain*. Springfield, Ill: Charles C. Thomas, Nov., 1951.
47. Worrell, Richard V. "Incidence of Chondoromalacia of Patella Following Menisectomy of Knee Joint," *New York State Journal of Medicine*, (1973).